Withdrawn
from
stock

# How to Drink Without Drinking

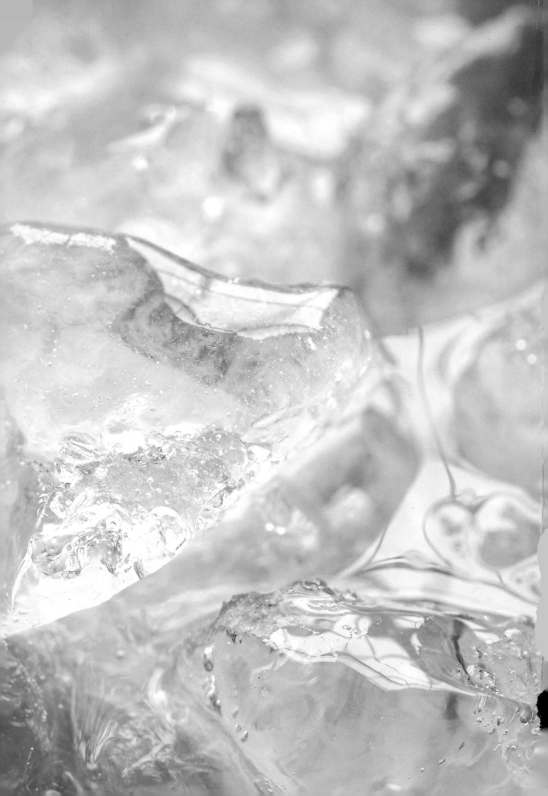

# How to Drink Without Drinking

*Celebratory alcohol-free drinks
for any time of the day*

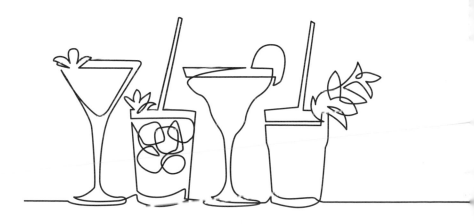

## Fiona Beckett

Photography by Nassima Rothacker

For Kate, Flyn and all my non-drinking friends

An Hachette UK Company
www.hachette.co.uk

First published in Great Britain in 2020 by
Kyle Books, an imprint of Kyle Cathie Ltd
Carmelite House
50 Victoria Embankment
London EC4Y 0DZ
www.kylebooks.co.uk

ISBN: 978 0 85783 6151

Distributed in the US by Hachette Book Group,
1290 Avenue of the Americas,
4th and 5th Floors, New York, NY 10104

Distributed in Canada by Canadian Manda Group, 664 Annette St.,
Toronto, Ontario, Canada M6S 2C8

Publisher: Joanna Copestick
Editor: Tara O'Sullivan
Editorial assistant: Sarah Kyle
Design: Rachel Cross
Photography: Nassima Rothacker
Food styling: Becks Wilkinson
Props styling: Cynthia Blackett
Production: Lucy Carter

A Cataloguing in Publication record for this title is available from
the British Library

Printed and bound in China

10 9 8 7 6 5 4 3 2 1

# CONTENTS

# INTRODUCTION

There's always been a significant minority of people who don't drink, but it's been growing exponentially, particularly among young adults. Over a quarter of 16–24 year olds – and half the world's population – don't drink at all for a variety of reasons, mainly religious and the desire to follow a more healthy lifestyle.

Others may take a temporary break when they're pregnant, unwell or taking a particular kind of medication, or abstaining for a period like Dry January or Sober October, for example.

Then there are those, including me, who do drink, not necessarily to excess, but like to take two or three days off a week to enjoy the added sharpness and focus of being clear-headed. It all adds up to a growing interest in, and market for, alcohol-free drinks.

Barely a day passes without some celeb or chef talking about how they've gone sober. Elton John, Rob Lowe, Russell Brand, Chris Martin of Coldplay, they're all out there testifying the difference it's made to their lives. Famous hard drinkers, like Dave McMillan of the legendary Joe Beef in Montreal, have been turned into born-again abstainers. There is even such a thing as a sober coach – someone whose job it is to keep A-listers on track.

For the rest of us, it's more similar to becoming flexitarian. We still eat meat, but not so much. We enjoy wine, but not every day. And that becomes progressively easier as more and more quality alcohol-free products come on to the market, and we learn to devise new and delicious drinks to replace the alcohol-based ones we're used to.

There's never been a better time to give up or cut down on booze, temporarily or permanently, and this book will show you how.

# HOW TO DRINK WITHOUT DRINKING

Just as with any lifestyle change, giving up alcohol, whether permanently or temporarily, needs a change of mindset. I'm obviously not talking about addiction issues here, for which you need professional help – as well as the realisation that you have a drinking problem – but simply choosing alcohol-free drinks rather than alcoholic ones.

You might think, earning my living by writing about wine, I'm the last person to advise you, but I see that as an advantage. Although I have to taste wine or other alcoholic drinks most days, like everyone else I benefit from a break from actually drinking them. But I'm not prepared to settle for second best. It's important to me that the days when I don't drink are as pleasurable in terms of what I consume as those when I do.

Only you will know whether you'll find it easier to cut alcohol out completely – even if for a limited period – or just drink on fewer occasions, but it pays to make a plan.

## 10 WAYS TO REDUCE (OR ELIMINATE) THE BOOZE IN YOUR LIFE

### 1. Set a personal goal
You have to start somewhere, but make it realistic. Two alcohol-free days a week is doable for most of us, most likely after the weekend. Three is better still – preferably in a row.

### 2. Don't make up for it on the days you drink alcohol
On some of the days when you are drinking, you might want to reduce the amount you drink to one drink a day, sipped slowly and mindfully rather than gulped unthinkingly. If you're trying to cut down, limit yourself to one (modest, not goldfish bowl-sized) glass with dinner or resolve not to drink when alone. Be aware and honest with yourself about what you're drinking when you do drink. An app may help you keep on track.

### 3. Tell your family and friends
Family should be on your side, but one of the biggest battles you'll face is friends who keep pressing you to drink, maybe implying that you've become a party pooper if you don't. Don't be

embarrassed to explain exactly why you're cutting down – or out – making it clear that you're serious. It may even involve changing your social circle. Find a non-drinking pal to go out with if the pressure's getting to you – a sobersister (or soberbro).

## 4. Don't needlessly put yourself in the way of temptation

On days or periods you're cutting down or cutting out, avoid your usual boozy haunts. Don't make having a drink the main reason for going out – unless it's a coffee.

In fact, it may be worth taking the car, which gives you an easy excuse not to drink. If you're embarking on a longer period of abstinence, clear out the booze from the cupboards and fridge and steer clear of the wine aisle. Stock up with alcohol-free alternatives instead (see pages 182–191).

## 5. B.Y.O. (Bring your own)

If you're visiting friends and are not sure if there will be something alcohol-free to drink, take it with you, particularly to a party. Alcohol-free beers, which look similar to the full-strength version, are an especially good bet as they won't make you stand out from the crowd. If you're away for the weekend, take a bottle of an alcohol-free spirit (see page 184) and some tonic to your hosts.

## 6. Think about food pairing

You're more likely to crave wine with food from wine-producing regions, especially Italy, France and Spain. So avoid the trattoria or tapas bar on your nights off in favour of your local Indian, Thai or Vietnamese. See pages 196–199 for my tips on pairing different cuisines with non-alcoholic drinks.

## 7. Get into alcohol-free cocktails

It's hard to find a substitute for wine, but alcohol-free cocktails can be mind-blowingly good these days, with many top restaurants offering an impressive selection. I often start the evening with one, whether I'm drinking or not, and end up drinking it with food.

## 8. M.Y.O. (Make your own)

There's a real pleasure and satisfaction in making your own drinks. Like home-cooked food, they taste so much better than the shop-bought version and are cheaper, too, making the best of seasonal produce (see Cordials and Shrubs, pages 26–49). Make them look as beautiful as they taste – be inspired by Nassima's gorgeous pictures in this book and serve them in lovely glasses and jugs. Indulge your senses.

## 9. Find another type of drink to get passionate about

Part of the appeal of wine, beer and other drinks like whisky, is the knowledge you accumulate about them – even working through a bucket list of drinks you want to try before you die. But you can apply that type of geekery to other drinks, too. Get into tea, get into coffee, get into fermenting – all fascinating, absorbing worlds.

## 10. Learn to love water

Probably your best friend on your sober days – or months – both on its own and as a chaser for any alcoholic drink you're drinking. (Don't drink because you're thirsty – drink for the taste.) Serve water cool, fresh and flavoured, if you like, with fruit, cucumber or herbs. (For more about water, see pages 19–23.)

## FOCUS ON THE PAY-OFFS

It's important to see alcohol-free days as an opportunity, not a deprivation. The proverbial glass half full rather than half empty. There are, as you'll rapidly discover, many advantages, even if you cut down rather than cutting out, including a better quality of sleep, improved concentration, weight loss (unless you binge on cakes instead), more spare cash and, due to the happy lack of hangovers, more productive hours in the day.

You may want to remind yourself of those benefits by writing them down or setting yourself a daily reminder on your phone.

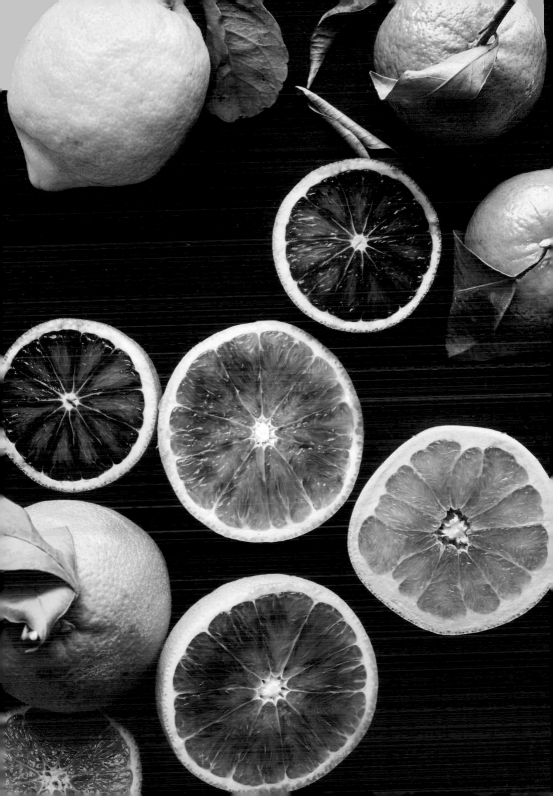

# THE ALCOHOL-FREE LARDER
*What You Need in Your Kitchen to Make Delicious Drinks*

A lot of the ingredients you'll need to make alcohol-free drinks will already be in your refrigerator and storecupboard, but it's worth accumulating one or two others, plus a few ready-made soft drinks you enjoy and regularly turn to.

## IN THE STORECUPBOARD
### Elderberry Juice
The most similar-tasting fruit juice to red wine.

### Flavoured Oils
Highly concentrated food-grade citrus oils can be used to boost citrus flavour without added sweetness. (You can achieve the same effect with bitters, but the result won't be entirely alcohol free – see page 16.) These are available from online ingredient suppliers such as souschef.co.uk.

### Flower Waters
Rose water and orange flower water, widely used in the Middle East, add an exotic touch to fruit juices.

### Long-life Dairy-free Milk
For making lattes and shakes (see pages 128–140).

### Mango Pulp/Purée
Available in cans from Indian and Asian grocery stores and some supermarkets, this is actually superior in flavour to fresh mango unless it's really ripe. Kesar mango pulp comes in 850g (1lb 14oz) cans.

### Passion Fruit Syrup
Again, more intense than fresh passion fruit, this is a versatile ingredient for cocktails.

### Lime Cordial
A good old-fashioned squash but still widely used by barmen on its own or to boost and round out the flavour of fresh lime.

### Spices
Juniper berries are invaluable if you want to make your own gin-style cordial,

such as my Juniper Syrup (see page 91). I'll add cardamom to practically anything. And mulling spices such as cinnamon, nutmeg and cloves can be used just as effectively in non-alcoholic drinks as alcohol-based ones (see Mulled "Wine" on page 99 and Mulled "Cider" on page 102).

## Sugar

Essential for making cordials and shrubs (see pages 26–49) and sugar syrup for cocktails (see page 14). Ordinary granulated sugar can be used in most cases.

## Teas and Tisanes

There's a vast range of fruit and herbal teas these days in addition to conventional black and green teas. Three of my favourites are rooibos tea, Turkish apple tea and dried lemon verbena (see page 167). These help avoid the urge to fall back on sugary drinks.

## Tomato Juice

An essential ingredient if you're a Virgin Mary fan (see pages 84–89).

## Verjus

A milder kind of vinegar made from unripe grapes, good for balancing a sweeter drink (see page 191).

## Vinegar

Especially raw cider vinegar, which is what you need for making shrubs (see pages 46–49). Other types of vinegar, such as wine vinegar and balsamic vinegar are useful for giving drinks a bit of an edge, but don't overdo it. And if you like a touch of tartness, fruit vinegars can be drunk diluted on their own.

# Sugar Syrup

This is the main weapon in the bartender's armoury, the point being to have
something to hand for sweetening your drinks that's as sweet as sugar but
without its grittiness. You can buy sugar syrup ready made, but the advantage of
a homemade version is that you can tailor it to your own taste. The classic way to
make it is to slowly dissolve sugar in an equal volume of water, but that does make
for an intensely sweet syrup. Increasingly I have experimented with using rather
less sugar, which affects the keeping quality slightly: full-strength sugar syrup
lasts a good month, a weaker solution maybe half to two-thirds that period of time.
Obviously it depends on the temperature of your refrigerator and the container you
keep it in, which should, of course, be scrupulously clean – I use a jam jar that has
been run through the dishwasher (see page 29).

You can vary the type of sugar you use – for example, using demerara sugar or dark
muscovado sugar instead of ordinary granulated sugar for making the syrup will
give your drinks more of a fudgy flavour.

### 1:1

Put 200g (7oz) granulated sugar in a pan with 200ml (7fl oz) cold water and heat over
a low heat, stirring occasionally, until all the sugar grains have dissolved. Bring to the
boil, then simmer for 1 minute without stirring. Take off the heat and leave to cool
completely before storing in a sterilized airtight container.

### 3:4

Make the syrup as above but reduce the quantity of sugar to 150g (5½oz) for a lighter
result.

### 1:2

Reduce the quantity of sugar further to 100g (3½oz) – good for longer drinks.

### Flavoured Syrups

It's easy to flavour your homemade sugar syrup – my own favourites are cardamom
syrup, made by adding about 10–12 lightly crushed cardamom pods to the syrup
once the sugar has dissolved and then straining out before storing, and Kaffir Lime
Syrup (see page 66).

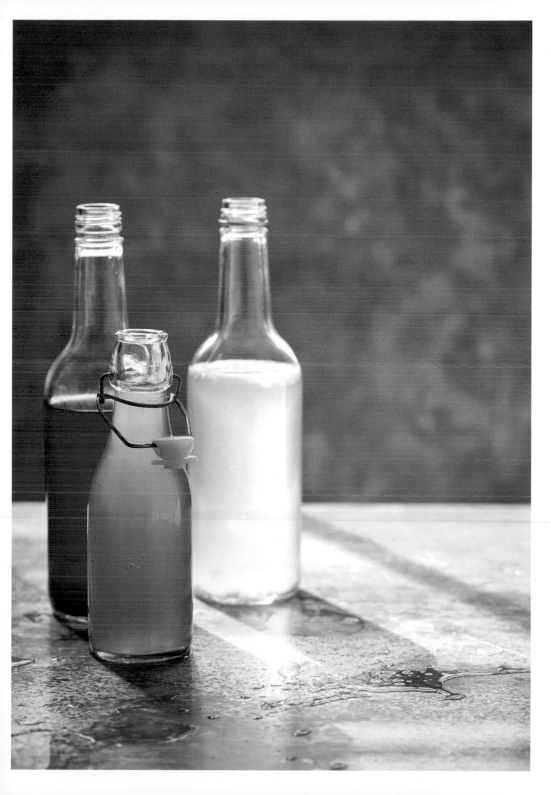

## IN THE REFRIGERATOR

### Fresh Dairy or Dairy-free Milk

For making lattes and shakes (though keep long-life back-ups in the storecupboard – see page 12). See page 189 for my favourite brands.

### Fresh Root Ginger

Adds zing to cordials and smoothies.

### Lemons and Limes

The most essential fresh ingredients for your drinks, preferably unwaxed in case you want to use the rind/zest.

### Seasonal Fruit

For making juices and smoothies (see pages 144–161).

## IN THE FREEZER

### Frozen Berries

Good for making cordials and shrubs (see pages 26–49) and shakes (such as my Frozen Raspberry, Coconut and Chia Shake, see page 140) when fresh berries are out of season, as well as for flavouring Kombucha (see page 116).

### Ice Cubes

You can never have enough (see Clean Ice, page 22).

## IN THE GARDEN

### Fresh Herbs

Rosemary and mint are especially useful.

### Lemon Verbena

Well worth growing and harvesting the fresh leaves, or drying and storing the leaves to make delicious French-style tisanes (see page 167).

## IN THE COCKTAIL CABINET

### Alcohol-free Spirits and Aperitifs

New examples are coming on to the market all the time, but at the time of writing the market leader is Seedlip (see page 184). A good base for "alt-gin" (as non-alcoholic gin is referred to) and tonic or to give cocktails a bit more depth and complexity.

### Bitters

With an ABV of 35–45%, you might think bitters are the last thing you want in an alcohol-free drinks cupboard, and indeed if you're trying to avoid alcohol altogether you should give them a miss. But if it's simply a question of trying to cut down on your alcohol consumption, bitters are used in such an infinitesimal quantity that they're going to make your drink no more alcoholic than an alcohol-free beer. And they do add flavour. The most well-known brand of bitters is Angostura.

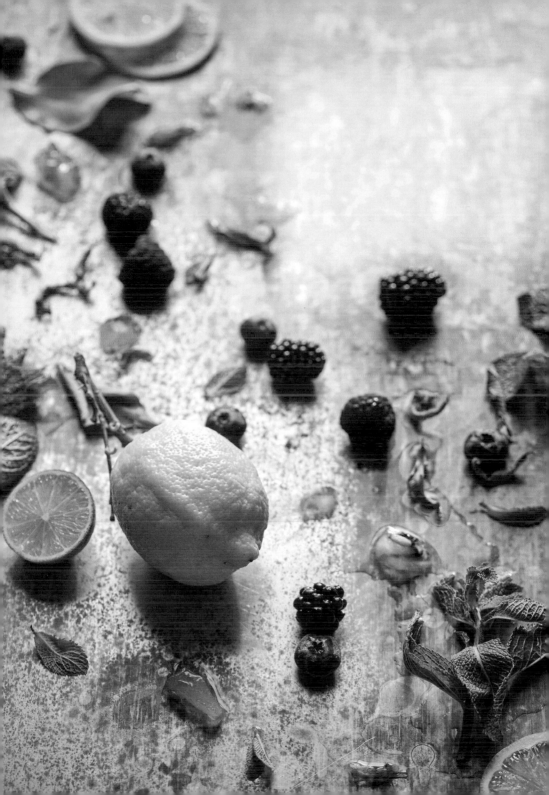

### Tonics and Other Mixers

Life has got a lot more complicated since the days when tonic water was synonymous with Schweppes. You used to be pretty confident your tonic water was Indian tonic water and that it would go with your gin (when you were drinking). Now it may be flavoured with all kinds of ingredients, which probably makes it a better drink to enjoy on its own.

*Tonic Water:* The classic Indian tonic water is flavoured with quinine, an ingredient derived from cinchona bark historically used for treating malaria. Its bitter flavour has a real affinity with the juniper in a London Dry gin, but is combined with citrus and a significant amount of sugar to make a palatable drink on its own. Schweppes currently has just under 5g (about a teaspoon) per 100ml (3½fl oz), while Fever-Tree has 7.1g (a heaped teaspoon) but no added artificial sweeteners. There are "slimline" and "light" tonics (no sugar in the case of Schweppes Slimline, 2.9g per 100ml in Fever-Tree Refreshingly Light).

There is also a vast range of flavoured tonic waters on offer, where Fever-Tree again leads the field. I always have their Aromatic Tonic Water and Mediterranean Tonic Water to hand (see Best Brands, page 185).

*Tonic Syrup:* This is favoured over tonic water by some bartenders as a purer form of quinine, to which you simply add soda water. It does admittedly make a more flavourful tonic drink, but it isn't that easy to get hold of.

*Soda Water:* Also known as club soda, this is sparkling water to which sodium bicarbonate has been added and is sugar free, which makes it ideal for diluting drinks that are already sweet or where you want to preserve the fresh fruit flavour, as in cordials and shrubs. You can also use sparkling water for the same purpose – see pages 26–49.

*Ginger Beer vs. Ginger Ale:* Much of a muchness in terms of taste, ginger beer is brewed, while ginger ale is a ginger-flavoured carbonated drink. It's rather more useful in the context of mixing drinks to know how sweet the product is (it's generally sweeter than tonic) and how fiery the ginger is – Devon producer Luscombe, for example, usefully produces both a cool and a hot ginger beer.

# WATER, WATER, EVERYWHERE...

You hardly need me to tell you that water is the obvious go-to for the non-drinker and drinker alike. We need it to keep our bodies functioning properly, and it's refreshing, cheap, easily available (except in parts of the world where clean water is tragically not) and has zero calories. In other words, it's the miracle drink.

## So What's the Problem?

Well, basically the taste. In modern industrial societies, the fact that tap water is heavily treated may be reassuring in one way, but one of the ingredients used in the process is chlorine, which has a distinct and not particularly pleasant flavour. Some sources, particularly in towns or in hard water areas, are more heavily treated than others. Drink water from the tap if you're on holiday in the Scottish Highlands, for example, and you'll be amazed how fresh and sweet it tastes.

## Should You Use a Water Filter?

One solution is to have a water filter, which will take the chlorine and traces of heavy metals out of the water that comes through your tap, or so the manufacturers say. Opinions differ on how effective or beneficial it is to filter water – you could write a whole book on the subject, never mind a paragraph – but for what it's worth, I find that using filtered water improves the taste of the drinks I make, especially tea and coffee. I also worry that although water is treated at source, it's still passing down ancient lead pipes to my tap and I'd rather not ingest the residues it is accumulating along the way. But do your own research – I'm not advocating you do the same, merely putting the issues out there.

## What About Mineral Water?

The other option is to buy bottled mineral water – or at least it was. It's definitely been dealt a blow by the shocking revelations of the extent to which plastic is polluting our seas and our water supplies. But you may still feel it's worth it to get water that is more to your personal taste and not chemically treated, particularly if you buy it in recyclable glass bottles.

As you'll know if you've experimented with them, mineral waters don't all taste the same because – no surprise here – of the different levels of minerals

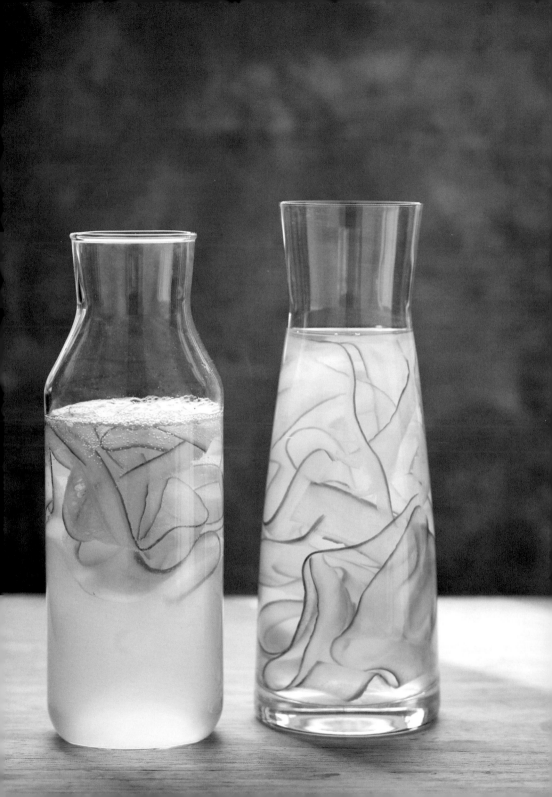

they contain. I like Evian and Perrier, for example, and dislike Fiji (too soft and sweet) and Badoit (too salty, containing 150mg sodium per litre compared to 9mg per litre in Perrier). It's worth taking a photo of the composition of a bottled water you like (you should find it on the back label – see below), then looking for waters that have similar levels of minerals.

Natural mineral water comes from specific underground water supplies, while spring water is taken from a single named source. In some cases, the water is naturally sparkling; in others pressurized $CO_2$ is added. Personally, I like sparkling water if I'm drinking it with fried food and seafood, and still water with meat, cheese and richer sauces, but there are, would you believe, water sommeliers who advise on the ideal pairings.

If you would like more specific information on bottled waters, check out the website finewaters.com.

*Reading Your Water Label:* You get far more information about bottled water than you do about wine. The back label will list such naturally occurring or added minerals as calcium, magnesium and potassium along with sodium, bicarbonates, sulphates, chlorides and nitrates. There should also be a figure for total dissolved solids (TDS) or dry residue, the total amount of minerals that are dissolved in the water – the higher the level, the more assertive the flavour. San Pellegrino, for example, has a TDS of 1,109mg per litre, Evian of 357.

### Flavoured Waters

I'm not a big fan of shop-bought flavoured water – it's just another source of sugar or artificial sweeteners and flavourings, and expensive to boot. But you can flavour your own quite simply by adding fresh herbs or fruit to it, as you may have spotted in the foyers and dining rooms of smart hotels. Fruit with a high water content, such as strawberries and melon, work particularly well, and so do citrus slices. Cucumber is also deliciously refreshing – long curls look sexier than slices – as are sprigs of rosemary, mint and lemon verbena (see Fresh Herbal Teas and Tisanes, page 166).

Sometimes you may prefer to drink your water hot, in which case lemon (reputed to be a system cleanser), rosemary and sage make ideal flavouring additions. There is no need for water to be boring.

### Tree Waters

Increasingly fashionable, tree waters, such as bamboo, birch and particularly coconut have made an appearance on the shelves of health and lifestyle shops and top-end department stores, the sell being that they're rich in antioxidants and minerals. Coconut water is admittedly quite distinctive (albeit high in sugar), but the rest to my mind are under-flavoured and overpriced – and you can get the same health benefits much more easily and cheaply from food.

### Clean Ice

Ice, like other ingredients in your refrigerator/freezer, can pick up odours from food. It also has a limited shelf life – if you leave it in an open tray or buy one of those gigantic bags of ready-made ice, there's a fair chance that the cubes will have acquired some off flavours by the time you finish it. Either way, it's best to decant ice cubes into small freezer bags so that you can keep them sealed and uncontaminated for as long as possible.

Purists among the bar-tending fraternity will also tend to make their ice with filtered or mineral water (I use filtered water myself).

In terms of the look of the ice, it's quite fun to make huge ice balls or, if it's just going to be tipped into a jug, large chunks of ice frozen in the cups of a muffin tin. You can also freeze decorative ingredients like fresh herbs, edible flowers, berries and quarter slices of citrus in the pieces or cubes of ice.

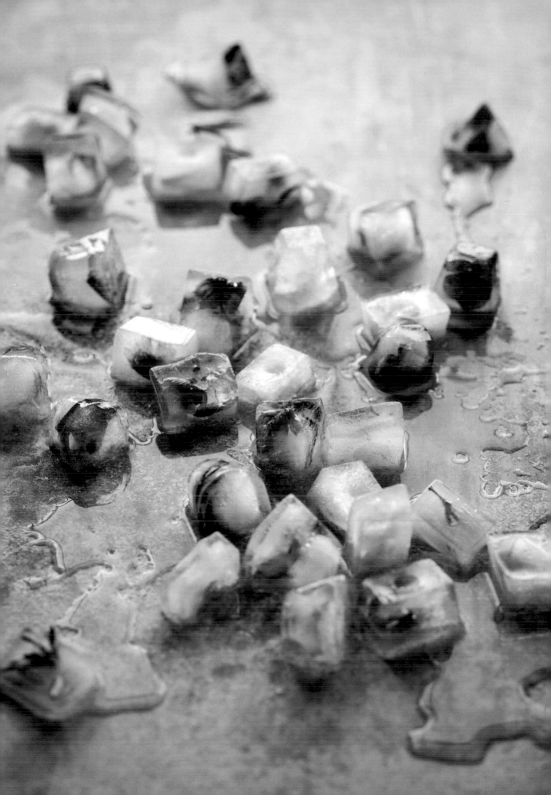

# Useful kit

You may very well have all the equipment you need in your kitchen to concoct delicious alcohol-free drinks, depending on what you want to make. But if you're embarking on fermented drinks like kefir or kombucha, for example (see pages 112–117), you'll need some large preserving jars. If juices and smoothies are more your thing, you'll need a powerful blender or food processor such as a NutriBullet, which will handily also crush ice.

The following items are those that I find most useful.

**Cocktail Measure, Measuring Jug and Measuring Spoons:** For obvious reasons. You may freewheel with your cocktails after a while, but to begin with I find it's best to go with the recommended proportions.

**Cocktail Shaker:** I just use a basic one, but if you're a perfectionist, some cocktails benefit from double straining. Fancy cocktail shakers have what they call a Hawthorne strainer (there are loads of videos on how to use them on YouTube), but I find a fine tea strainer, which you can pick up for a fraction of the price, does the job perfectly well. Just remember to rinse it immediately after use, otherwise you can never get the bits out of it.

**Disposable Gloves:** Unglamorous but hugely useful for handling ingredients that may otherwise stain your hands such as turmeric and beetroot.

**Funnels:** In general, I find it easier to fill a bottle without splashing sticky syrup all over my work surface by using a jug and a funnel. You may need a smaller and a larger one depending on the size of the bottle neck.

**Glass Bottles:** Essential for storing your drinks in the refrigerator, but bear in mind that you may run out of tall storage space in the door. I found the 250ml (9fl oz) lidded glass milk bottles from Lakeland particularly useful, as they fit on an internal shelf. Small bottles are nice to give as presents, too – IKEA and Wilko are good hunting grounds, or snap them up in the sales.

**Preserving Jars:** These jars, such as Kilner or Mason jars, are not cheap, but are essential if you're into fermenting (see pages 108–123). Note that you may need to buy replacement rubber seals after a while.

**Fine Sieve:** For straining off fruit from a cordial (see pages 28–49). You can alternatively use a colander lined with muslin.

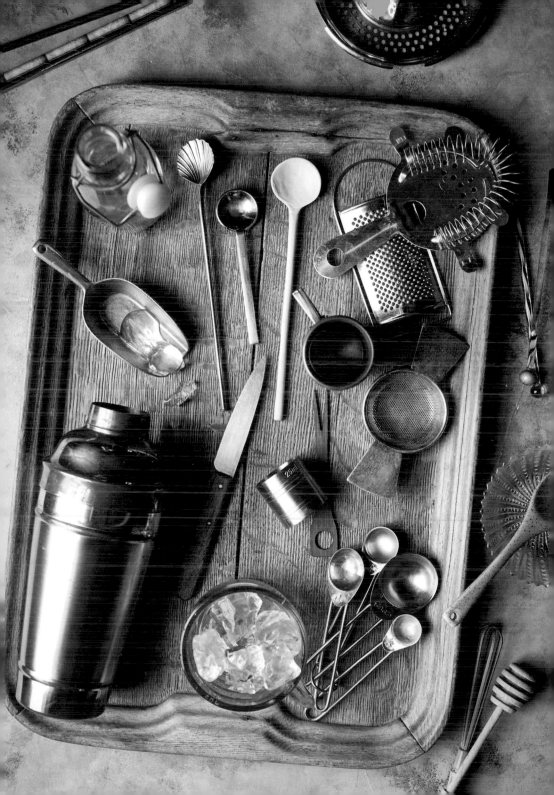

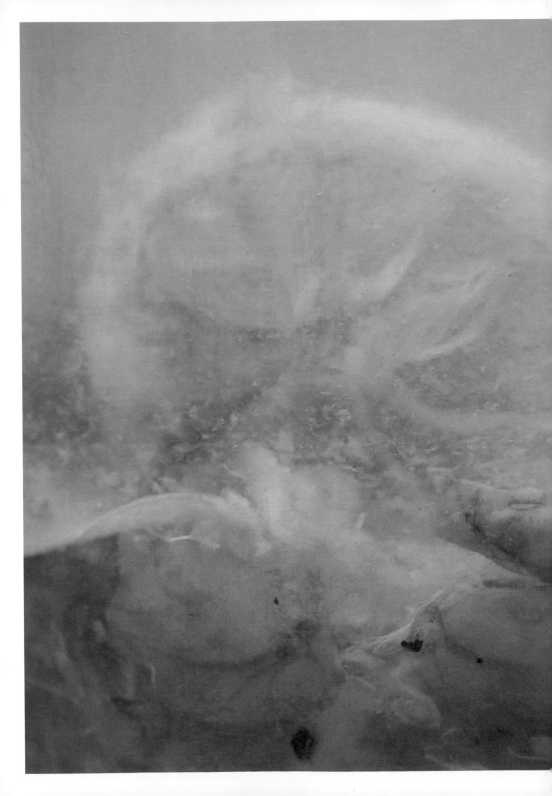

# CORDIALS
# AND SHRUBS

Cordials and shrubs should be at the heart of your alcohol-free larder if you want fresh, natural-tasting drinks. Personally, I like to keep them seasonal rather than make them to last for months. I don't want to drink cherry-flavoured drinks in mid-winter any more than I want to eat a cherry pie. Like homemade ice cream, they're best not designed to keep for months.

The two drinks are actually very similar – cordials are made from fruit and sugar or sugar syrup, while shrubs add vinegar to that. They are more tart, obviously, and take slightly longer to make as the vinegar needs time to integrate with the sugar and the fruit.

Drinking vinegar goes back to Greek and Roman times but had a renaissance in the 19th century, when "switchels" became popular in the US, consumed by agricultural workers out in the fields. (Try the home-made version on page 45).

I like the idea of foraging for your cordials and shrubs. Elderflower is the obvious choice for the early summer (much improved by gooseberries which come into season about the same time). Wild cherries, which I was given by a friend from his allotment last year, are a revelation, with so much more flavour than the commercially grown variety. Quince, despite the pain of peeling them, is almost an equal favourite, making a beautiful pink-gold drink. The more frugally minded among you can even use the peelings – and, I discovered, citrus shells, to make a "fruitstock", which won't be as intense as a cordial, but makes a gently refreshing drink. It's obviously better to do this with organic or home-grown fruit.

If you're making a cordial or shrub, think about whether you'll get a more intense flavour if you cook the fruit. With soft or semi-soft fruits, it's generally not necessary – blackberries being an exception – but sharp or hard fruit, like gooseberries, cranberries, quince and rhubarb, all taste better cooked, in my opinion.

Finally, remember that your cordial is like a squash or shop-bought cordial and not intended to be drunk neat. Dilute them to taste with sparkling water or, in the case of shrubs, soda water. I generally like about 1 measure of cordial to 4 measures of water or mixer, though sometimes the cordial is just so delicious I can't resist having it a little stronger.

# How to sterilize a bottle

Even if you want to keep a drink for a relatively short time, it's important your container is scrupulously clean. I don't want to encourage you to be sloppy about hygiene, but I generally find a run-through on the dishwasher is enough to achieve that so long as the bottle has been thoroughly cleaned as soon as you've used up the previous contents (for which it will help to buy a bottle brush). If you don't have a dishwasher, the bottle won't fit, or the top is too narrow to ensure you can clean it thoroughly, you need to wash and rinse it by hand, then place the open bottle on a baking sheet and place it in the oven at 180°C/350°F/gas mark 4 for 10 minutes. Remove and let cool before use.

# CORDIALS

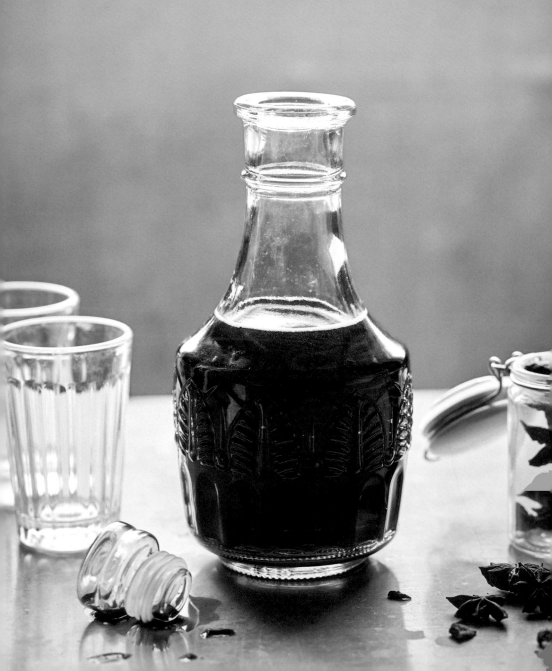

# Wild Cherry and Star Anise Cordial

Wild or sour cherries have a lovely tart flavour and a beautiful deep colour that makes a stunning-looking summer drink, one of my favourites in the book. Obviously it depends how many wild cherries you can get your hands on – you don't need to work exactly to this recipe, just roughly these proportions. If you can't find wild cherries you could use other fresh cherries when in season or frozen cherries at a pinch, but the flavour won't be quite as wonderful.

**MAKES ABOUT 600ML (20FL OZ)**

600g (1lb 5oz) ripe wild cherries
1 whole star anise, or equivalent in broken pieces
about 250g (10½oz) granulated sugar (you need just over half the quantity of liquid)
soda or sparkling water, to serve

Pick over the cherries, removing the stalks and discarding any damaged or broken ones. Tip into a colander, rinse and then weigh the fruit.

Transfer the cherries to a saucepan, cover with water and add the star anise. Bring gradually up to boiling point, then simmer for about 15 minutes.

Remove the star anise, then strain the liquid through a fine sieve into a large measuring jug, pressing down on the cherries to break them and extract their juice. Check the quantity of liquid – I ended up with 500ml (18fl oz) – and pour back into the pan. Add the sugar and heat over a low heat, stirring occasionally, until it has completely dissolved. Bring to the boil, then simmer for 2 minutes.

Take off the heat, skim off any froth on the surface and leave for 10 minutes to settle. Pour the cordial through a funnel into a sterilized bottle. Seal, cool and store in the refrigerator for up to 2 weeks. Alternatively, freeze in plastic tubs for up to 3 months.

To serve, dilute to taste with soda or sparkling water.

# Christmas Cranberry Cordial

You can, of course, buy cranberry juice everywhere, but this has a much more intense flavour and a vivid scarlet colour that will make you feel fabulously festive. You can save the strained-off fruit and use it as a topping for muesli, stir it into porridge or add it to a fruit loaf or teabread.

**MAKES ABOUT 600ML (20FL OZ)**

250g (9oz) granulated sugar
400ml (14fl oz) water
200g (7oz) cranberries, rinsed
2 finely pared strips of unwaxed orange or clementine rind
piece of cinnamon stick
30ml (2 tablespoons) freshly squeezed orange or clementine juice, strained
soda or sparkling water, to serve

Put the sugar in a saucepan and add the measured water. Heat over a low heat, stirring occasionally, until the sugar has completely dissolved. Bring to the boil and add the cranberries, orange or clementine rind and cinnamon. Simmer for 5 minutes until the skins of the cranberries have split but the berries are still holding their shape. Take off the heat, add the orange or clementine juice and leave to cool.

Strain the contents of the pan through a fine sieve into a wide-necked jug or bowl, then pour the liquid through a funnel into a sterilized bottle or other airtight container, seal and leave in the refrigerator for 24–48 hours before using; it will keep for up to 2 weeks in the refrigerator.

To serve, dilute 4:1 or 5:1 with soda or sparkling water.

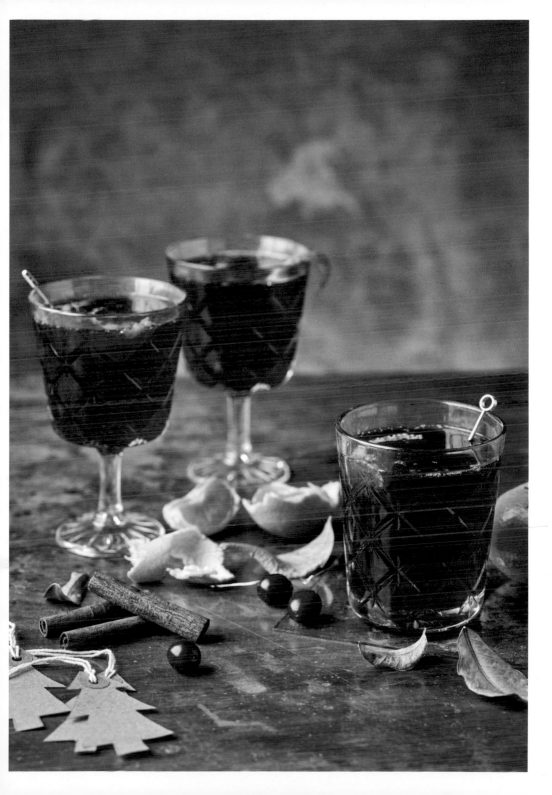

# Quince, Honey and Lemon Cordial

Quince makes the most beautiful pale golden pink cordial, perhaps the prettiest of them all. I was going to make a shrub with it (see page 46), but the flavour was so heavenly it seemed a shame to take away from it. It also leaves you with a delicious compote that you can enjoy on its own or as the basis of a pie or crumble.

**MAKES ABOUT 1 LITRE (1¾ PINTS) CORDIAL,** *PLUS 4–6 SERVINGS OF QUINCE COMPOTE*

1kg (2lb 4oz) quinces – 5–6 medium-sized fruit, about 750g (1lb 10oz) peeled weight
1.5 litres (2¾ pints) water
500g (1lb 2oz) granulated sugar
75g (2¾oz) clear honey (or agave syrup)
thinly pared rind of 1 small unwaxed lemon
soda or sparkling water, to serve

Peel, core and cut up the quinces (save the trimmings to make the Quince and Lemon Fruitstock on page 41).

Pour the measured water into a large saucepan and add the sugar and honey or agave syrup. Heat over a low heat, stirring occasionally, until the sugar has completely dissolved. Add the lemon rind and bring to the boil. Tip in the quince and bring back to the boil, then reduce the heat, partially cover the pan and simmer for about an hour or until the fruit is soft.

Strain the contents of the pan through a fine sieve into a wide-necked jug or bowl. Transfer the poached quince to a separate bowl with a little of the liquid to moisten the fruit. Then pour the remaining juice through a funnel into sterilized bottles. Seal, leave to cool and store in the refrigerator for up to 2 weeks.

To serve, dilute to taste with soda or sparkling water.

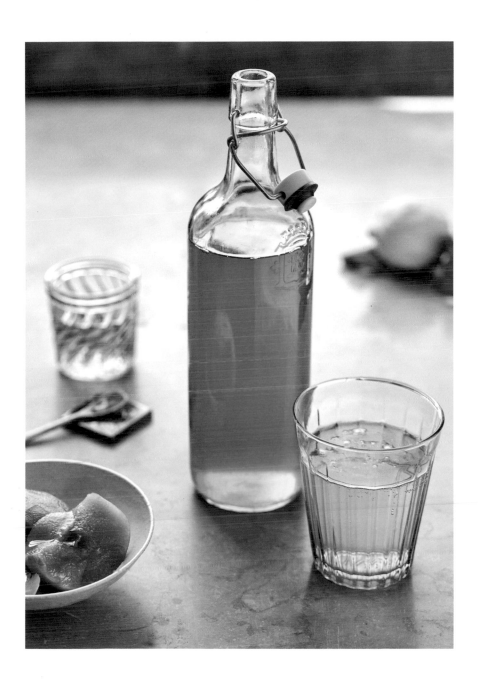

# Gooseberry and Elderflower Cordial

With their delicate creamy-coloured blossoms, elderflowers are so pretty and pleasurable to harvest – the essence of summer. Pick them early on a fine day, not when it's been raining, and use them as quickly as possible. You can make the cordial without citric acid if you're not intending to keep it for long, but don't overdo the lemon, otherwise it will just taste like lemonade.

**MAKES 1.5 LITRES**
**(2¾ PINTS)**

10–12 freshly picked heads of elderflower (or more if you pick smaller florets)
600g (1lb 5oz) granulated sugar
600ml (20fl oz) water
250g (9oz) green gooseberries, topped and tailed
2 unwaxed lemons, or 1 unwaxed lemon and 20g (¾oz) (maybe less) citric acid
soda or sparkling water, to serve

Pick over the elderflower heads, trimming the flowers away from the stalk and shaking out any insects.

Put the sugar in a large saucepan and add the measured water. Heat over a low heat, stirring occasionally, until the sugar has completely dissolved. Bring to the boil and add the gooseberries. Simmer for 7–8 minutes, then take off the heat.

While the gooseberries are simmering, finely pare the rind of the lemon(s) and slice the flesh. Swirl the elderflowers gently in a bowl of cold water.

Remove the elderflowers from the water and add to the sugar syrup along with the lemon rind and slices and the citric acid, if using. Stir, lightly cover with a clean tea towel and leave in a cool place overnight.

Strain the cordial through a fine sieve into a wide-necked jug or bowl. Pour the cordial through a funnel into 2 x 75cl) sterilized glass bottles and seal. Store in the refrigerator and consume within a month. You can also freeze the cordial in plastic bottles, though remember to leave some headspace to allow the liquid to expand.

To serve, dilute to taste with soda or sparkling water.

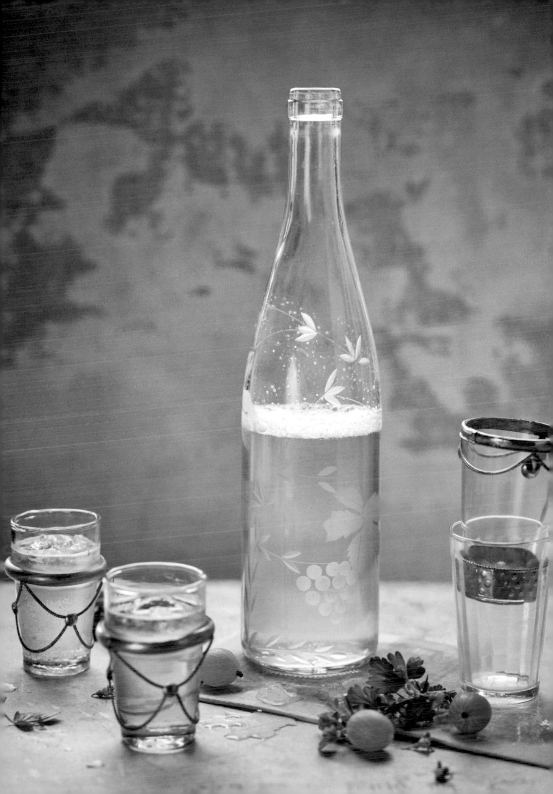

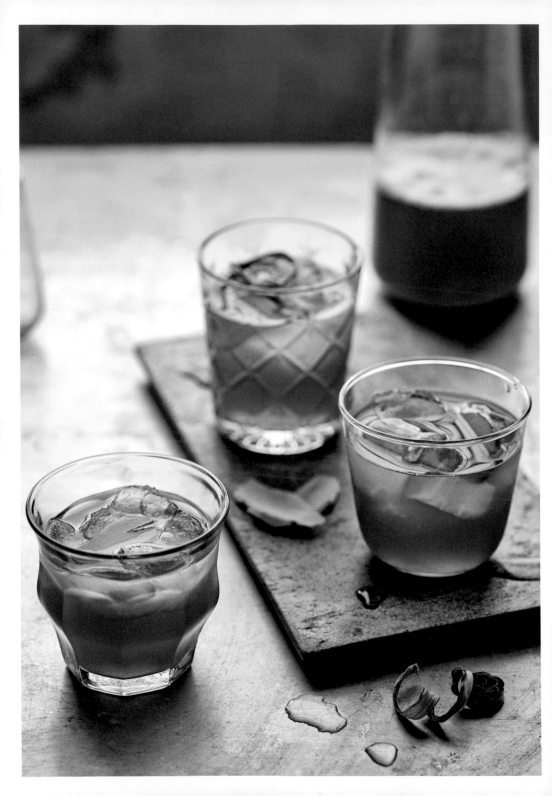

# Rhubarb Cordial

I often felt before writing this book that it was a waste not to use the marvellous juice from poaching rhubarb, particularly the pretty pale pink forced rhubarb you get at the beginning of the season. Just add a little extra water and you have a delicious drink, which I've kept a bit tarter than some of the other cordials in order to show off the flavour of the fruit (or vegetable, as it should strictly be considered).

**MAKES ABOUT 450ML (16FL OZ) CORDIAL,**
*PLUS 4 SERVINGS OF POACHED RHUBARB*

450g (1lb) rhubarb, ideally
  the early-season pink
  forced variety
100g (3½oz) caster sugar
slice of fresh root ginger
finely pared strip of
  unwaxed lemon rind
250ml (9fl oz) water
Sugar Syrup (see page 14),
  to sweeten if you find that
  it's too sharp
soda water or ginger ale
  and ice (optional), to serve

Trim the rhubarb stalks and cut into chunks, then put into a medium–large saucepan. Tip over the sugar, add the ginger and lemon rind and pour over the measured water. Heat over a low heat and bring slowly up to simmering point, stirring occasionally. Cover and simmer for about 6–7 minutes until the fruit is almost soft but not broken up. Take off the heat and leave to infuse for about 30 minutes.

Tip the contents of the pan into a fine sieve over a bowl and leave to strain for an hour or so. Taste the juice and add sugar syrup to sweeten if you like (but bear in mind that if you add a mixer it will sweeten the cordial slightly, too). Transfer the poached rhubarb to a bowl with a couple of tablespoons of the juice to moisten. Then pour the remaining juice through a funnel into a sterilized bottle or other airtight container, seal and refrigerate. It will keep for up to 2 weeks in the refrigerator.

To serve, pour into tumblers with or without ice and top up with soda water or (particularly good) ginger ale.

# FRUITSTOCK

*It occurred to me one day that there was no reason to let the peelings left over from preparing fruit go to waste. Here are three ways to make a waste-not-want-not fruitstock from discarded fruit peelings and/or squeezed citrus shells. Although I've written these as recipes, feel free to adjust the quantities depending on the peel and shells you have available.*

## Apple Lemonade

I made this on impulse when I was writing a book called *The Frugal Cook* and discovered it was absolutely delicious.

**MAKES ABOUT 500ML (18FL OZ)**

leftover peelings from 2 large Bramley apples or 3–4 smaller apples
shells of 1 large or 2 smaller unwaxed lemons
Sugar Syrup (see page 14), to taste

Put the apple peelings and lemon shell(s) in a saucepan and pour over enough water to cover. Bring to the boil, then simmer for 20 minutes or so.

Strain the contents of the pan through a fine sieve into a wide-necked jug or bowl and sweeten to taste with sugar syrup. Leave to cool, then pour through a funnel into a sterilized bottle, seal and store in the refrigerator for up to 2 weeks.

To serve, dilute with water to taste.

# Quince and Lemon Fruitstock

This isn't as refined as the cordial made with the peeled fruit (see page 34), but quinces are rare and it does give you a second bite at the cherry, as it were…

**MAKES ABOUT 1 LITRE (1¾ PINTS)**

leftover quince peelings from Quince, Honey and Lemon Cordial (see page 34)
2 unwaxed lemon shells
1 litre (1¾ pints) water
granulated sugar
raw apple cider vinegar (optional – if turning it into a shrub)

Put all the quince peelings and lemon shells in a saucepan, pour over the measured water and bring to the boil. Simmer for about an hour.

Take off the heat and strain the contents of the pan through a fine sieve into a large measuring jug. Check the quantity of liquid, pour back into the pan and add one-third the quantity of granulated sugar to liquid. Heat over a low heat, stirring occasionally, until the sugar has completely dissolved. Bring to the boil, then simmer for 2 minutes. Take off the heat and leave to cool. Pour the Fruitstock through a funnel into sterilized bottles, seal and store in the refrigerator for up to 2 weeks.

To turn this into a shrub (see page 46), once the Fruitstock is cool, stir in about one-third the quantity of raw apple cider vinegar to the liquid you measured in the measuring jug. Transfer to a sterilized large preserving jar or bottles, allowing about 2–3cm (approx. 1 inch) of headspace, seal and leave in a cool place for a week or so to mature, then transfer to the refrigerator where it will keep for up to 2 weeks.

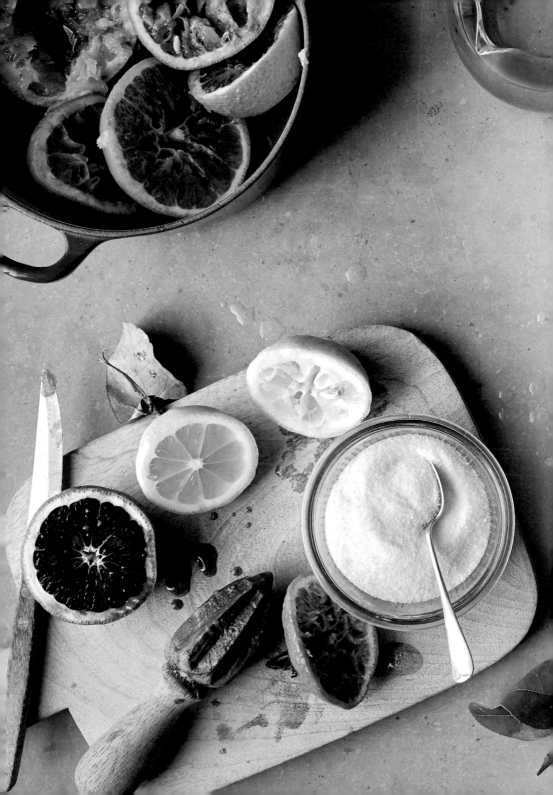

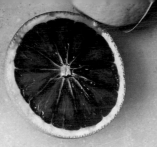

# Paddington Syrup

This makes a slightly bitter marmalade-tasting syrup, which I've called Paddington Syrup for obvious reasons. . .

assortment of unwaxed citrus shells, such as sweet orange, ruby grapefruit and lemon – whatever you've been using (grapefruit and lemon will obviously make the syrup rather more bitter)
granulated sugar
tonic water, ginger ale or ginger beer, to serve

Put the citrus shells in a saucepan, cover with water and bring to the boil, then simmer for 30–40 minutes. Take off the heat and leave to infuse for 30 minutes.

Remove the shells, squeezing them to extract any remaining juice. Strain the liquid through a fine sieve into a large measuring jug. Check the quantity, pour back into the pan and add half the quantity of granulated sugar to liquid. Heat over a low heat, stirring occasionally, until the sugar has completely dissolved. Bring to the boil, then simmer for 2 minutes. Take off the heat and leave to cool.

Pour the syrup through a funnel into sterilized bottles, seal and store in the refrigerator for up to 2 weeks.

To serve, dilute the syrup with tonic water, ginger ale or ginger beer to taste.

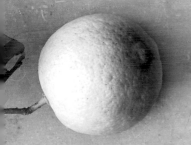

# Bergamot Lemonade

Bergamot is the wild child of the citrus world. Rare, exotic and fragrant, it lifts lemonade to another plane. I couldn't stop drinking this when I made it, though you may want to add a little extra sugar if you don't like your drinks too tart. You can, of course, make this with unwaxed lemons instead.

**MAKES 500ML (18FL OZ)**

3 unwaxed bergamots
150–175g (5½–6oz) caster sugar
500ml (18fl oz) boiling water
slices of cucumber, slices of bergamot or lemon and a sprig of mint, to garnish
water or cold-infused tea (see below), to serve

Very finely pare the rind of the bergamots, leaving the white pith behind.

Juice the fruit and put in a heatproof bowl or jug along with the rind and sugar. Pour over the measured boiling water and stir until the sugar has dissolved. Cover the bowl with a clean tea towel and leave to infuse for 3–4 hours.

Strain the mixture through a fine sieve into a wide-necked jug or bowl.

To serve, dilute with a little water or cold-infused tea (see below) and garnish with cucumber and bergamot or lemon slices and a sprig of mint. Any remaining lemonade can be stored in a sterilized bottle in the refrigerator for 2–3 days.

---

### VARIATION: EARL GREY LEMONADE

*Bergamot is the ingredient that's used to flavour Earl Grey tea, so adding tea to this lemonade is a natural step. What you need is a cold-infused light black tea – something like Darjeeling or a light oolong. Simply add 3 tea bags or heaped teaspoons of tea leaves to a teapot or heatproof jug, pour over 400ml (14fl oz) cold water and leave for 3–4 hours to infuse (about the same time as the lemonade takes). Then add the tea to your lemonade to taste – go steady, as you don't want it to overwhelm the bergamot.*

# Switchel

I hadn't heard of switchel before I wrote this book. It's a type of shrub, of Caribbean origin – also known as Haymaker's punch – that found its way into rural America where it would be drunk by the workers in the fields. It's much more enjoyable than drinking cider vinegar on its own. Adjust the quantities to your own personal taste.

SERVES 2

1–2 teaspoons (5–10g) grated fresh ginger
3 tablespoons raw cider vinegar
2–3 tablespoons maple syrup or raw honey
1 teaspoon freshly squeezed lemon or lime juice
400ml (14fl oz) still or sparkling water, plus extra water to dilute

Add all the ingredients to a sterilized wide-necked bottle or jar and cover with the lid. Give it a shake, taste, adjusting the sweetness, and refrigerate for 24 hours.

Strain through a fine sieve and pour into glasses, adding extra still or sparkling water to taste.

# SHRUBS

*Shrubs are made by adding vinegar – usually apple cider vinegar, which is less sharp than wine vinegar – to fruit and sugar. You can make them with fresh fruit, as in the strawberry shrub here, or with cooked fruit, which works better with fruits like blackberries, plums and rhubarb, which need warming to bring out their flavour.*

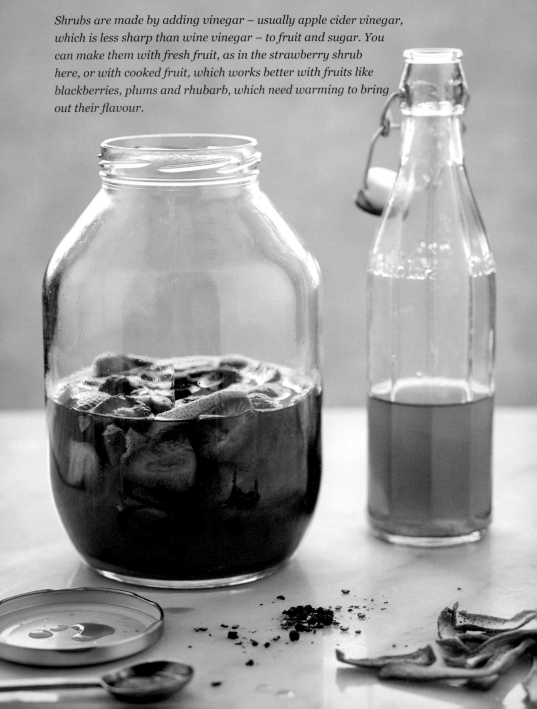

# Strawberry and Roasted Orange Shrub

Drinks writer Kate Hawkings, co-owner of the Bellita Bar in Bristol, UK, taught me how to make shrubs. Strawberries make a particularly good shrub. Kate uses black pepper in her version, but I like the added touch of roasted orange rind, strawberries having a natural affinity with orange.

**MAKES ABOUT 1.4 LITRES (2½ PINTS)**

500g (1lb 2oz) ripe strawberries, hulled and halved or quartered, depending on size
350g (12oz) granulated sugar
1 unwaxed orange
1 teaspoon black peppercorns, lightly crushed
500ml (18fl oz) raw apple cider vinegar
still or sparkling water, to serve

Put the prepared strawberries in a sterilized 2-litre (3½-pint) preserving jar with the sugar and stir well. Seal and leave in a cool place for 24–36 hours until the sugar has dissolved, giving it a stir halfway through.

To roast the orange rind, preheat the oven to 180°C/350°F/Gas Mark 4. Line a baking sheet with nonstick baking paper.

Finely pare the rind of the orange, scatter over the lined baking sheet and bake for 10–12 minutes until crisp and fragrant. Remove from the oven and let cool.

Add the roasted orange rind and lightly crushed peppercorns to the preserving jar, pour in the vinegar and stir together. Scrunch a piece of nonstick baking paper into the top of the jar to keep the fruit submerged, loosely close the preserving jar lid and leave in a cool place for about 10 days. Taste it after a week – it should be tart but not unpleasantly so.

Strain the liquid through a fine sieve into a wide-necked jug or bowl, then pour through a funnel into 2 x 75cl sterilized glass bottles and seal. It will keep – and continue improving in flavour – for about 2–3 weeks in the refrigerator.

To serve, dilute to taste with still or sparkling water.

# Blackberry and Cinnamon Shrub

When you pick blackberries, you may normally think of a pie or a crumble, but save enough to make this delicious shrub as well. Although you can turn raw soft fruits into a shrub, I love the extra flavour you get from cooking blackberries and it integrates better with the cinnamon.

**MAKES ABOUT 600ML (20FL OZ)**

250g (9 oz) granulated sugar
250ml (9fl oz) water
450–500g (1–1lb 2oz) blackberries
¼–½ teaspoon ground cinnamon
200ml (7fl oz) raw apple cider vinegar
sparkling water or apple juice and sparkling water, to serve

Put the sugar in a saucepan and add the measured water. Heat over a low heat, stirring occasionally, until the sugar has completely dissolved. Bring to the boil and add the blackberries and cinnamon, then simmer for 10–12 minutes until the blackberries are soft.

Take off the heat and leave to macerate for about 15 minutes. Tip the contents of the pan into a fine sieve over a bowl and leave to strain, then press down gently on the berries to extract their juice. Stir the vinegar into the liquid, then pour it through a funnel into a sterilized bottle, seal and leave in the refrigerator for at least 24–48 hours; it will keep for 2–3 weeks in the refrigerator.

To serve, dilute 4:1 or 5:1 with sparkling water or half apple juice and half sparkling water.

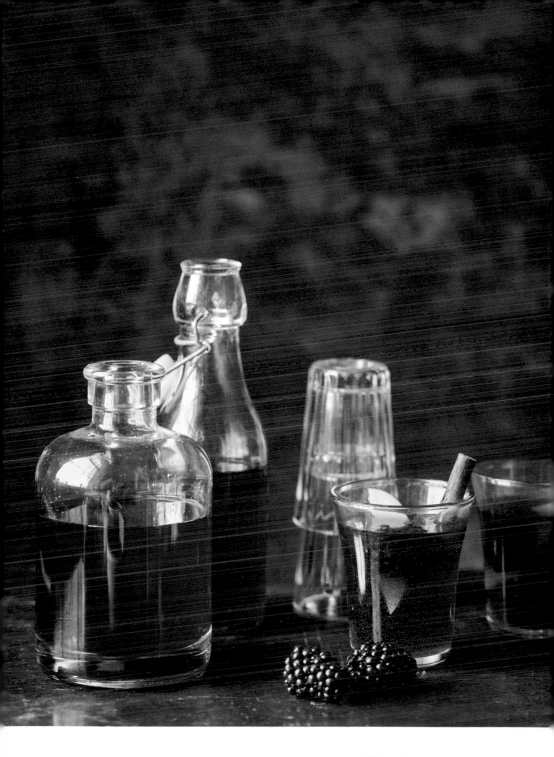

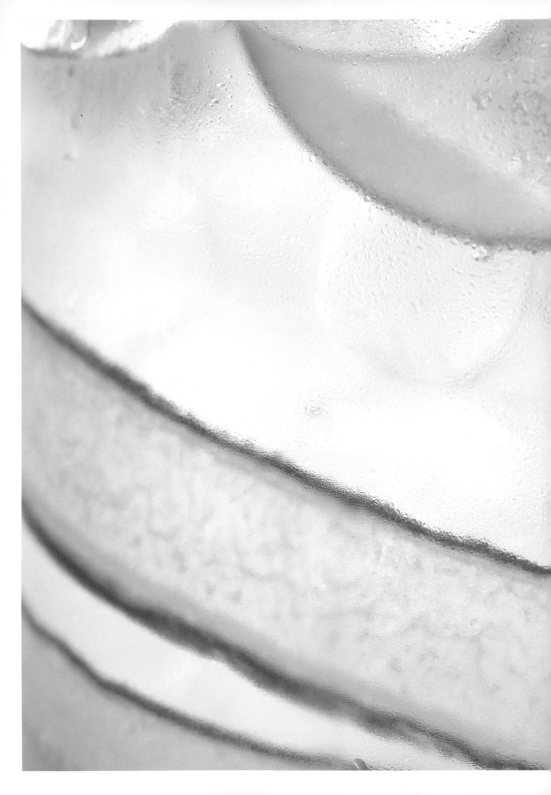

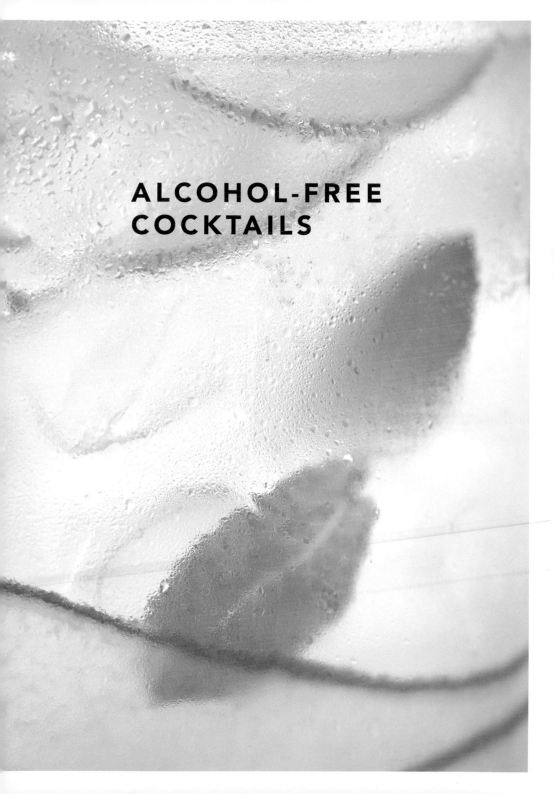

# ALCOHOL-FREE
# COCKTAILS

While it's possible to whip up a delicious alcohol-free cocktail (sorry, but I loathe the word "mocktail"), some cocktails adapt to a lack of booze better than others. A vodka-less Virgin Mary or a rum-free Piña Colada, for example, can be just as good as the full-strength version.

The main problem, if you don't have a particularly sweet tooth, is to stop them tasting too sickly. The strength of alcohol counteracts the sweetness of other ingredients in many cocktails. Take that away and you can be left with a drink that is cloying rather than refreshing. You may want to have a slightly heavier hand than usual with the lemon and lime, and grapefruit can add a welcome touch of bitterness. Tea, which I've used in the Strawberry "Pimm's" (see page 80) and the Long Island Iced Tea (see page 71), can add structure and tannin, too.

More complicated cocktails that normally involve more than one kind of alcohol are more challenging. I've yet to find the perfect Negroni, Manhattan or Martini. You just won't without the booze, although I have to admit that the Aecorn range of aperitifs, which was released just as I finished writing this book (see page 184) may be a game changer.

There are plenty of other products, however, to help you on your way, with more coming out all the time. Alcohol-free spirits mimic gin quite successfully, though as they are made in many different styles and with different ingredients, are not as usefully interchangeable, and some will work better for some cocktails than others. You do need to adapt and play around.

The French firm Monin makes a huge range of alcohol-free syrups, including a gin flavour, triple sec syrup and blue curaçao, that you can buy online (see page 186).

If you're creative, you can also make delicious drinks at home. What alcohol-free cocktails lack in strength they can make up for in freshness and natural fruit flavours. When I was developing the recipes for this book, I just added ingredients one by one, tasting until I got it right, then doubled, trebled or quadrupled them to make them in larger quantities.

Sometimes it didn't take multiple ingredients. The Lychee Martini (see page 56), for example, is good with an alcohol-free spirit (Ceder's in this case), but could be as simple as pouring chilled lychee juice into a frosted martini glass. Presentation is hugely important in terms of making you feel you're having a "proper" drink.

On the whole I've tried to keep things simple, imagining that you, like me, don't want to spend hours pretending you're a top mixologist. That's what we all go to cocktail bars for, right? But take inspiration from them and recreate the flavours at home – just as you would if you were trying to make a restaurant dish you'd been impressed by.

# Breakfast Martini

This is an alcohol-free version of one of my favourite cocktails, British steakhouse and cocktail bar Hawksmoor's Marmalade Cocktail. You need more marmalade than you do with the gin-based version (not a bad thing), and a couple of drops of orange oil or bitters really boost the flavour.

**SERVES 1**

1 tablespoon Seville orange
   (i.e. bitter) marmalade
50ml (2fl oz) Seedlip Spice
   94 or other alcohol-free
   gin alternative
50ml (2fl oz) freshly
   squeezed orange juice
20ml (4 teaspoons) freshly
   squeezed lemon juice
15ml (1 tablespoon) Sugar
   Syrup (see page 14)
handful of ice cubes
2 drops of orange oil or
   bitters (optional)

Spoon the marmalade into a cocktail shaker, pour in the Seedlip Spice 94 or other alcohol-free gin alternative and stir. Add the orange and lemon juices, sugar syrup and ice and shake vigorously.

Taste, adding a couple of drops of orange oil or orange bitters if you want to intensify the orange flavour.

Strain into a martini glass and serve.

*VARIATION: BUCKS FIZZ*
*You can use the Breakfast Martini as a base for a great Bucks Fizz. Make as above, divide between two Champagne flutes and top up with chilled alcohol-free sparkling wine.*

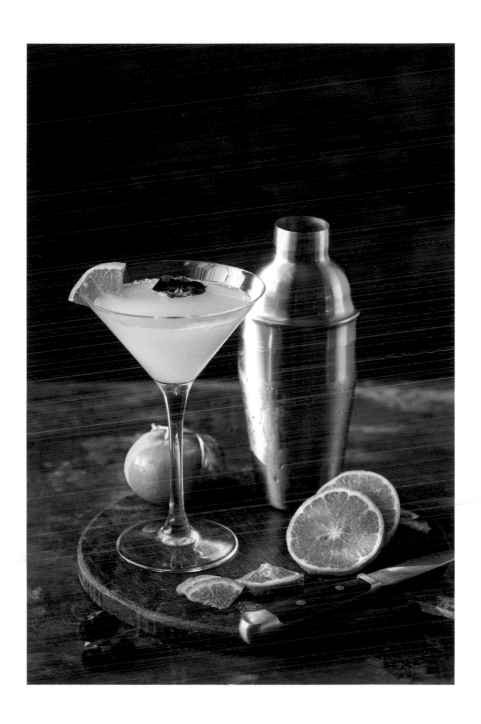

# Lychee Martini

It might look incredibly sophisticated but this cocktail is so simple it hardly deserves to be called a recipe. You can even make it without the alcohol-free spirit if you can find a good enough lychee juice (I like the Rubicon brand). But it really is so pale, pretty and delicious that you should definitely give it a go.

**SERVES 1**

ice cubes
25ml (scant 1fl oz) Ceder's Classic or other alcohol-free gin alternative
100ml (3½fl oz) lychee juice (I use Rubicon)
5ml (1 teaspoon) freshly squeezed lemon juice
a few drops of Hibiscus Syrup (see page 170) or Rhubarb Cordial (see page 39) for colour (optional)
edible flowers (optional) and 1 canned lychee, to garnish

Fill a cocktail shaker with ice, add all the ingredients except the garnish and shake vigorously.

Strain into a martini glass. Cut the lychee almost in half and slide down on to the rim of the glass to garnish, then serve, sprinkled with edible flowers (if using).

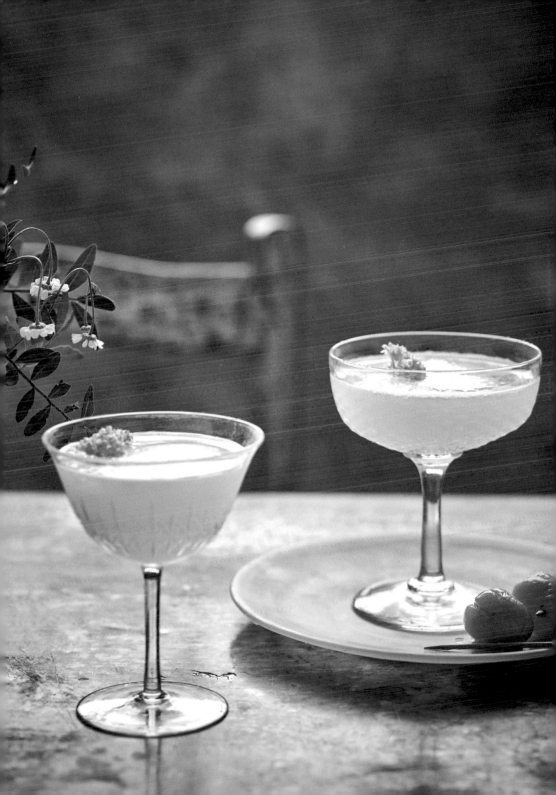

# Frozen Strawberry and Watermelon Margarita

Strawberry and watermelon is a great combination even without the tequila of a classic Margarita, though you could add a shot or two of alcohol-free vodka, if you like. Obviously it's best made in summer when both strawberries and watermelon are ripe – the perfect drink to sit and sip in the garden. You don't have to add salt to the rim of your glass – it's equally delicious without.

**SERVES 1**

1 fresh lime, halved
sea salt flakes (optional)
handful of ice cubes
175g (6oz) strawberries,
   hulled and halved, plus an
   extra slice to garnish
175g (6oz) watermelon,
   peeled, deseeded and cut
   into chunks
Sugar Syrup (see page 14),
   to taste (optional)
basil, to garnish

Juice half the lime. To salt the rim of your glass, wipe the cut surface of the other lime half around the rim of each glass, then dip into a saucer of sea salt flakes.

Crush the ice cubes in a powerful blender, or wrap them in a clean tea towel and smash with a rolling pin if your blender isn't powerful enough.

Add the strawberries and watermelon chunks and 1 tablespoon of the lime juice to the crushed ice in the blender and whizz until you get a frozen slush. Check for sweetness, adding extra lime juice or sugar syrup to taste if needed, then pour into a chilled martini glass. Garnish with a basil leaf and a slice of strawberry.

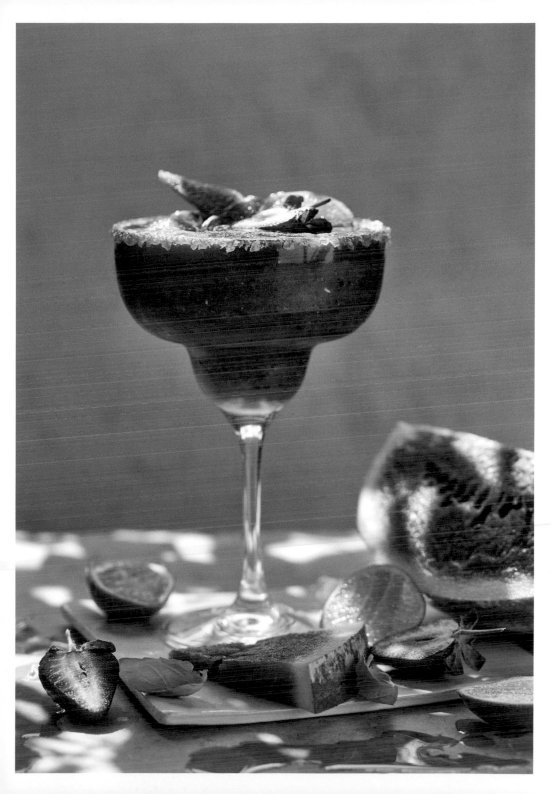

# Hibiscus and Rose Cosmopolitan

A Cosmo is classically made with cranberry juice, but I've found that you can just as easily substitute hibiscus syrup made from dried hibiscus flowers – see the Hibiscus Agua Fresca recipe on page 170. They have the same vivid colour as cranberries but a lovely floral aroma, too.

**SERVES 1**

ice cubes
60ml (4 tablespoons)
   Hibiscus Syrup (see page
   170)
30ml (2 tablespoons) freshly
   squeezed orange juice
15ml (1 tablespoon) freshly
   squeezed lime juice
splash of pink lemonade (the
   French La Mortuacienne is
   a good one)
2 drops of rose water
orange twist or poached
   hibiscus flowers (reserved
   from making the Hibiscus
   Syrup), to garnish

Fill a cocktail shaker with ice, add all the ingredients except the garnish and shake vigorously.

Strain into a martini glass, garnish with an orange twist or 1–2 of your poached hibiscus flowers and serve.

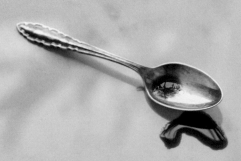
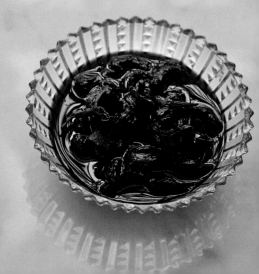

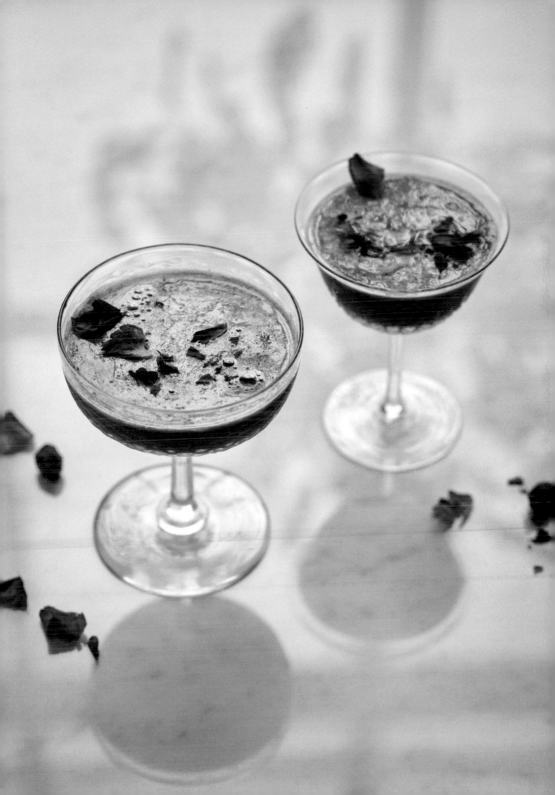

# St Clement's Punch

For a long time this has been my go-to for a New Year's Day brunch. Given the probable lateness of the night before, you might not feel like juicing all the fruit, particularly if you're doubling up and making it for a crowd, so it's fine to use a high-quality chilled ready-squeezed juice (not made from concentrate). I personally like to add a dash of Grand Marnier, which deepens the flavour without making it particularly alcoholic, but you can use an alcohol-free triple sec syrup like Monin, too. *Pictured on page 65.*

SERVES 6

500ml (18fl oz) freshly
squeezed orange juice
300ml (10fl oz) freshly
squeezed pink grapefruit
juice
500ml (18fl oz) homemade
or real lemonade
30ml (2 tablespoons) Monin
Triple Sec Curaçao syrup,
Grand Marnier or other
orange-flavoured liqueur
(optional, see above)
slices of orange, lemon and
pink grapefruit, to garnish

Pour the orange and pink grapefruit juices into a jug, top up with the lemonade and stir well.

To give the punch an extra edge, add the alcohol-free triple sec syrup or, if you don't mind a very small amount of alcohol, the Grand Marnier or other orange-flavoured liqueur.

Add a few slices of orange, lemon and pink grapefruit to the jug to garnish and serve.

# Passionate Lady

White Lady is one of those classic perfectly balanced cocktails that is hard to replicate. The original contains two kinds of booze, gin and Cointreau or triple sec, so although passion fruit syrup makes a pretty good substitute, you do need something orangey with it, too, hence the citrusy Seedlip Grove 42. You can also make a vegan version using a little aquafaba – the liquid drained from a can of chickpeas – instead of raw egg white. *Pictured on page 64.*

## SERVES 2

100ml (3½fl oz) Seedlip Grove 42 or other alcohol-free gin alternative
50ml (2fl oz) passion fruit syrup
50ml (2fl oz) freshly squeezed lemon juice
1 very fresh egg white or 15ml (1 tablespoon) aquafaba
handful of ice cubes
2 twists of finely pared unwaxed lemon rind, to garnish

Pour the Seedlip Grove 42 or other alcohol-free gin alternative into a cocktail shaker with the passion fruit syrup, lemon juice and egg white or aquafaba, and shake vigorously. Add the ice and shake again.

Strain into two chilled martini glasses and garnish each with a strip of lemon rind.

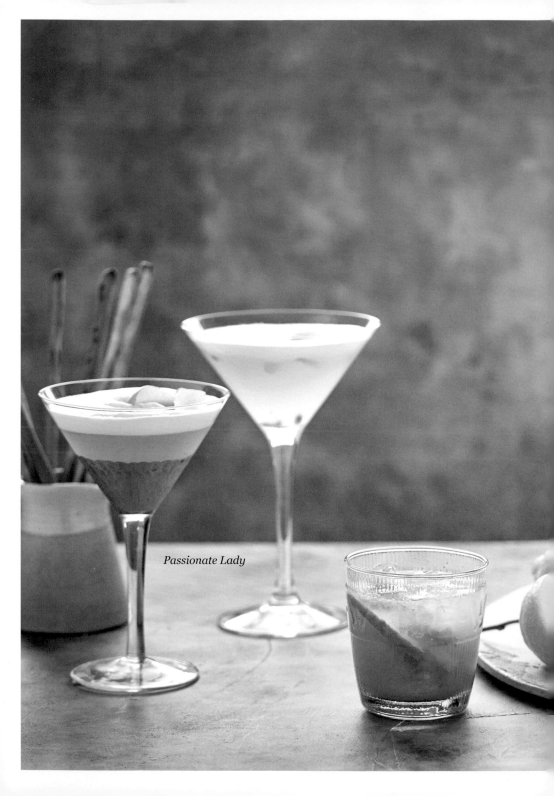

*Passionate Lady*

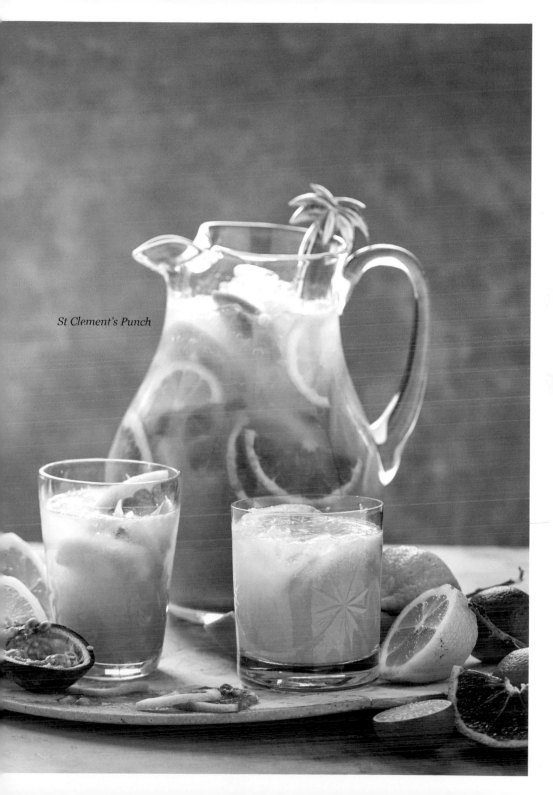

*St Clement's Punch*

# Kaffir Lime Syrup

Besides using in the Kaffir Lime Mojito opposite, you can enjoy this simply diluted with still or sparkling water to taste. *Pictured on page 69.*

**MAKES 300ML (10FL OZ)**

3–4 kaffir limes
200g (7oz) granulated sugar
300ml (10fl oz) water

Using a vegetable peeler, finely peel the rind of the kaffir limes, taking with it as little of the white pith as possible. Juice the limes and set aside.

To make the syrup, put the sugar in a saucepan and add the measured water. Place over a low heat, stirring occasionally, until the sugar has completely dissolved. Bring to the boil and add the lime rind, then simmer for 3 minutes. Take off the heat and leave to cool.

Stir in the lime juice, then strain the syrup through a fine sieve into a wide-necked jug or bowl. Pour through a funnel into a sterilized bottle or jar, seal and store in the refrigerator for up to 2 weeks.

# Kaffir Lime Mojito

Kaffir limes are wonderfully fragrant in comparison to ordinary limes – a bit like a bergamot is to a lemon – and they more than make up for the lack of rum in this classic cocktail. If you can't find fresh kaffir limes, you can use the more widely available frozen ones, but the flavour of the rind is not quite so intense. I suggest garnishing with a wedge of ordinary lime, though, because the pith of kaffir limes is so thick. *Pictured on page 68.*

**SERVES 1**

about 10 mint leaves, plus 1
    sprig to garnish
pinch of coarse sea salt
2 x 30ml (2 tablespoon)
    shots of Kaffir Lime Syrup
    (see opposite)
wedge of lime
crushed ice
chilled soda water, to top up

Put the mint leaves in the bottom of a wide, heavy-based tumbler, sprinkle over the salt and lightly crush with a muddler or the end of a rolling pin. Pour in the kaffir lime syrup, then squeeze over the wedge of lime, drop it into the glass and stir.

Fill the glass halfway with crushed ice, top up with chilled soda water and stir. Garnish with a sprig of mint and serve.

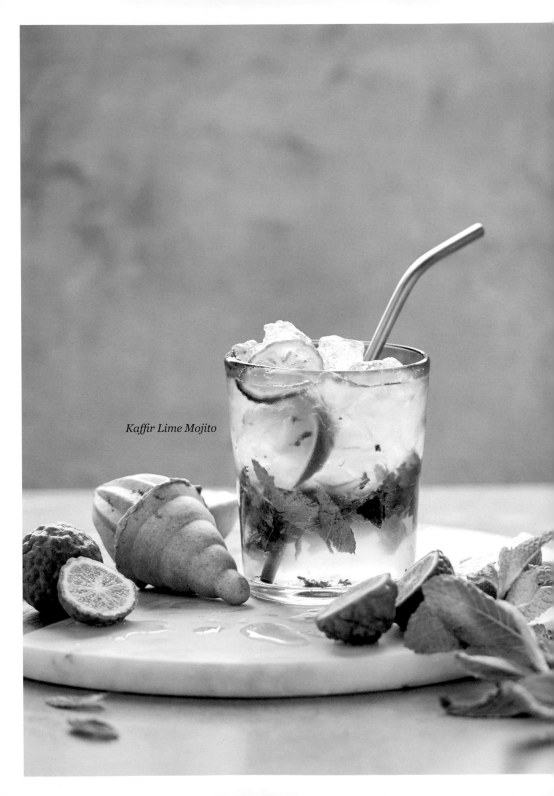

*Kaffir Lime Mojito*

*Kaffir Lime Syrup*

# Double Lime and Soda

A refreshing non-alcoholic version of one of the simplest cocktails out there, the Gin Rickey. I like to use Rose's Lime Cordial instead of sugar syrup to boost the fresh lime flavour. It makes quite a sharply flavoured drink, so you may want to add some basic Sugar Syrup (see page 14) to sweeten. You could also add a dash of Seedlip Garden 108 if you have some to hand.

SERVES 1

juice of 1 lime
equal quantity of Rose's
 Lime Cordial
4–5 ice cubes
chilled soda water, to top up
2–3 slices of lime, to garnish

Pour the lime juice into a tumbler and add the lime cordial. Drop in the ice cubes and stir.

Top up with chilled soda water, garnish with the slices of lime and serve.

# Lemonade and Ginger Beer Shandy

Perfect for a hot afternoon, this is possibly one of the easiest drinks to make, the exact proportions being dependent on the lemonade and ginger beer (or ginger ale) you use. Although this recipe serves 1–2 people, it's simple enough to increase the quantities to make a jug drink.

SERVES 1–2

150ml (5fl oz) chilled
 premium cloudy lemonade
100ml (3½fl oz) chilled
 ginger beer (or ginger ale)
1–2 slices of lemon

Pour the lemonade into a large glass (or two glasses, if making for two). Top up with the ginger beer (or ginger ale), stir and drop in the slice or slices of lemon, then serve.

# Long Island Iced Tea

The irony is that although Long Island Iced Tea sounds like a non-alcoholic drink, it's anything but. The original contains rum, gin, vodka, tequila and triple sec. In fact, it's absolutely lethal. The only ingredient my alcohol-free version shares with it is Coca-Cola, which, along with strong black tea, is key to the flavour of the finished drink. Though I say it myself, this is rather delicious.

**SERVES 4–6**

3 good-quality breakfast
  tea bags
500ml (18fl oz) boiling water
Original (not Diet) Coca-
  Cola
clear lemonade (use one of
  the good-quality brands
  made with real lemon)
5ml (1 teaspoon) passion
  fruit or peach syrup, or to
  taste
Sugar Syrup (see page 14),
  to taste (optional)
dash of Angostura bitters
  (optional)
ice cubes
3–4 slices of lemon and a
  sprig of mint, to garnish

Put the tea bags in a large measuring jug and pour over the measured boiling water. Leave to brew for 5 minutes, then remove the tea bags without squeezing them (you don't want to extract the bitter tannins). Leave the tea to cool.

Measure how much tea there is and add an equal quantity of Coke and one-third the quantity of lemonade, then stir to mix. Add the passion fruit or peach syrup to taste, plus a little sugar syrup if you don't find it sweet enough. You can also add a dash of Angostura bitters, if you like.

Fill a large jug with ice cubes and pour over the tea mixture, then add the slices of lemon and sprig of mint to garnish and serve.

# Sea Breeze

A simple two-ingredient version of the popular 1970s cocktail that tastes just as good without the vodka. Despite its summery vibe, the fresh ingredients are most likely to be available through the winter, so think of it as a cheering shot of sharp bright citrus through the dark days of December and January. I like it made with pink or ruby grapefruit juice, which is sweeter than the yellow variety, so you don't need to add sugar syrup to it (though obviously do if you feel it needs it – see page 14). Do make it with freshly squeezed grapefruit juice, though. You can shake it with ice in a cocktail shaker, but I'm perfectly happy to drink it over ice.

**SERVES 2**

ice cubes
freshly squeezed juice of 1
   pink or ruby grapefruit,
   about 150ml (5fl oz),
   strained
equal quantity of cranberry
   juice, e.g. about 150ml
   (5fl oz)
2 slices of lime, to garnish

Fill 2 tumblers with ice. Mix the grapefruit and cranberry juices together and pour over the ice.

Garnish each drink with a slice of lime and serve.

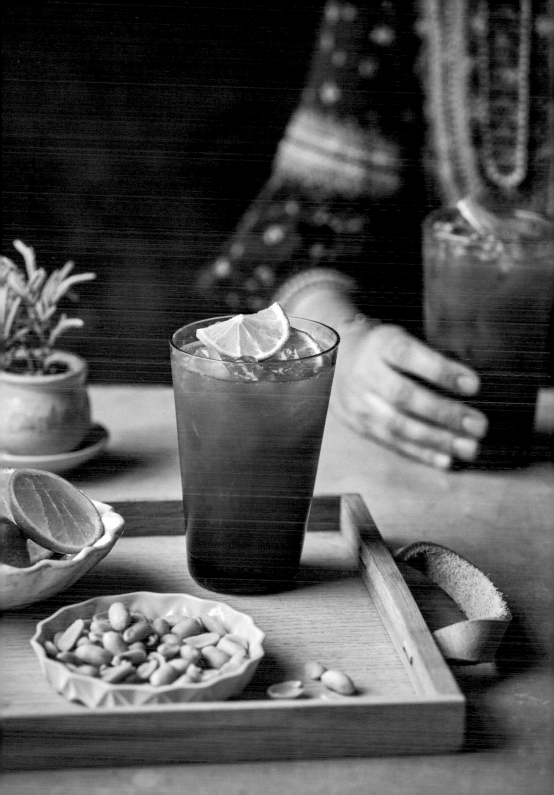

# Piña Colada

I made this a couple of times and couldn't get it pineappley enough or creamy enough to make up for the lack of rum. The solution I found – unless you're lucky enough to get your hands on a really ripe pineapple – is to make it with the pineapple cubes in fruit juice that you can buy in pouches (Dole makes them) or even canned pineapple. It obviously makes the drink quicker to prepare, too. *Pictured on pages 76–77.*

**SERVES 4**

400g (14oz) pouch or can pineapple, about 220g (8oz) drained weight but reserve the juice
300ml (10fl oz) canned light coconut milk
2 unwaxed limes
2 handfuls of ice cubes, about 150g (5½oz) in total
30–45ml (2–3 tablespoons) light agave syrup
coconut water or Water Kefir (see page 114), optional

Drain the pineapple cubes, setting aside the juice. Open the can of coconut milk and give it a good stir, then measure out your 300ml (10fl oz). Juice one of the limes – you should get 45ml (3 tablespoons) juice – and have the other to hand with a Microplane grater.

Crush the ice cubes in a powerful blender, or wrap them in a clean tea towel and smash with a rolling pin if your blender isn't powerful enough.

Add the pineapple cubes to the/a blender with the crushed ice and blend until smooth. Pour in the coconut milk, lime juice and 30ml (2 tablespoons) each of the pineapple juice and agave syrup, and blend again. Add extra agave syrup to taste and enough extra liquid to make an easy drinking consistency – the liquid could be more pineapple juice, or a splash of coconut water or water kefir.

Divide between 4–6 chilled martini glasses and grate a little lime zest over each glass.

# Speightstown Sour

Caribbean supermarkets have loads of cordials on offer if you want an alcohol-free drink. My favourite on a recent trip to Barbados was the tamarind syrup, which does duty for a rum punch. You should be able to buy it in Caribbean grocery stores back home or order it online. *Pictured on pages 76–77.*

**SERVES 1**

ice cubes
25ml (scant 1fl oz) tamarind
  syrup
sparkling water, to top up
wedge of lime

Fill a glass with ice. Pour over the tamarind syrup, top up with sparkling water (about 4:1) and stir. Squeeze over the wedge of lime and drop it into your drink, then serve.

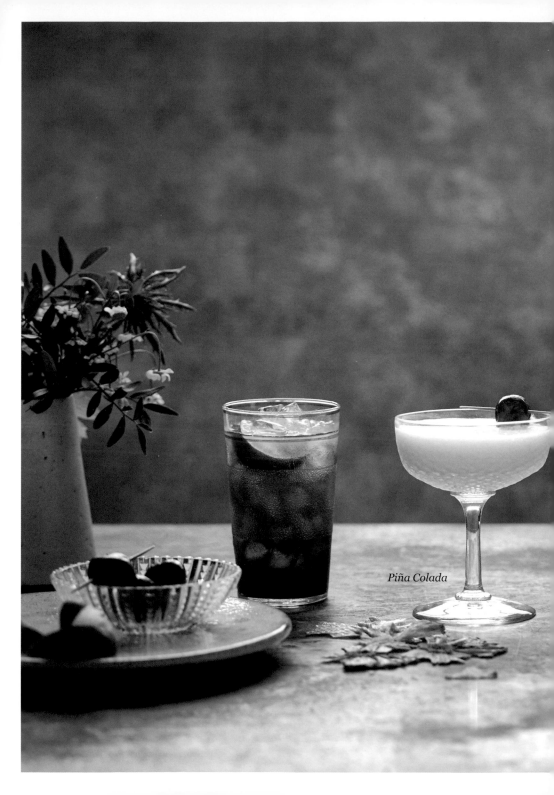

*Piña Colada*

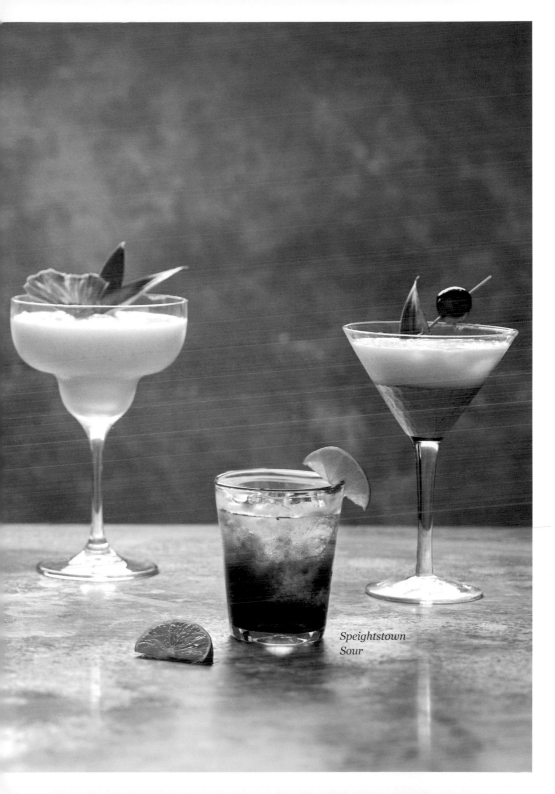

*Speightstown
Sour*

# Mai Tai

Mai Tai is classified as a Tiki – a Pacific island-style tropical drink that used to be popular back in the 1960s. It's still fun to serve right now with wildly kitsch accessories like umbrellas and swizzle sticks – you can't really go over the top with a tiki (just Google "tiki garnish"). Note that you will need some specialist ingredients for this one, including Caleño, a Columbian-inspired alcohol-free spirit flavoured with inca berries, or other rum substitute, and orange and almond syrups (I used Monin), all of which you can buy online. And it's quite a bit sweeter than the other cocktails, which may or may not be to your taste.

## SERVES 1

crushed ice
50ml (2fl oz) Caleño (see recipe introduction) or other alcohol-free rum alternative
juice of ½ unwaxed lime, about 25ml (scant 1fl oz), shell reserved
25ml (scant 1fl oz) Triple Sec or Curaçao syrup (e.g. Monin)
25ml (scant 1fl oz) Almond (Orgeat) syrup
25ml (scant 1fl oz) freshly squeezed orange juice

Fill a cocktail shaker with crushed ice, add the Caleño or other alcohol-free rum, lime juice, curaçao and almond (orgeat) syrups and orange juice. Shake well.

Pour the drink, crushed ice included, into a large tumbler, tucking the lime shell into the drink. Garnish like crazy with, say, an umbrella and a plastic palm tree, and serve with a straw.

# Hurricane

Another tiki, this time with passion fruit as the dominant note. I've used passion fruit syrup for ease and intensity of flavour, but use fresh passion fruit if you can lay your hands on some sufficiently ripe ones, in which case you may need a little Sugar Syrup (see page 14) to boost the sweetness. If you want to make it slightly less sweet, add a squeeze of lemon juice as well as the lime.

**SERVES 1**

ice cubes
50ml (2fl oz) Caleño
(see page 184) or
other alcohol-free rum
alternative
50ml (2fl oz) freshly
squeezed orange juice
25ml (1fl oz) passion fruit
syrup
25ml (1fl oz) freshly
squeezed lime juice
12.5ml (2½ teaspoons)
freshly squeezed lemon
juice (optional)
12.5ml (2½ teaspoons)
grenadine syrup
2 slices of orange and a
maraschino cherry, to
garnish

Fill a cocktail shaker with ice, add all the ingredients except the garnishes and shake vigorously.

Pour into a Hurricane glass if you have one or a tumbler if you don't. Garnish with the slices of orange and maraschino cherry and serve.

# Strawberry "Pimm's"

If you miss your Pimm's in the summer months, I promise you this is at least as good if not better. Stick to strawberries – you won't miss the other fruit. Note that you will need to brew the tea and macerate the strawberries in advance.

**SERVES 4–6**

2 breakfast tea bags
300ml (10fl oz) cold water
250g (9oz) strawberries
1 tablespoon caster sugar
15ml (1 tablespoon)
  balsamic vinegar
700ml (1¼ pints) clear
  lemonade (use one of the
  good-quality brands made
  with real lemon)
generous handful of ice
  cubes
2 sprigs of mint, to garnish

Put the tea bags in a jug, pour over the measured water and leave to infuse for 2 hours.

Meanwhile, hull the strawberries, removing any unripe white fruit around the stalk, and slice thickly. Put in a shallow dish and sprinkle with the sugar and vinegar. Turn the fruit over with a tablespoon and leave to macerate while the tea infuses.

Fish the tea bags out of the jug, add the strawberries with their juice and the lemonade and stir to mix. Add the ice cubes, garnish with the sprigs of mint and serve.

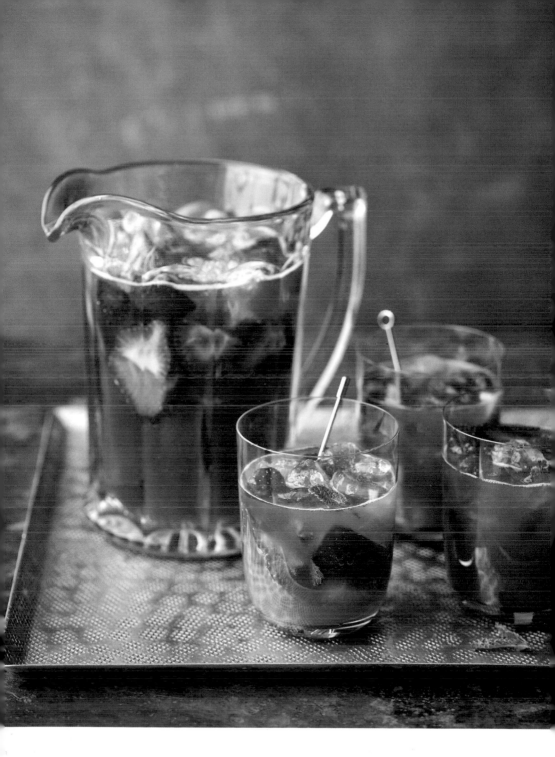

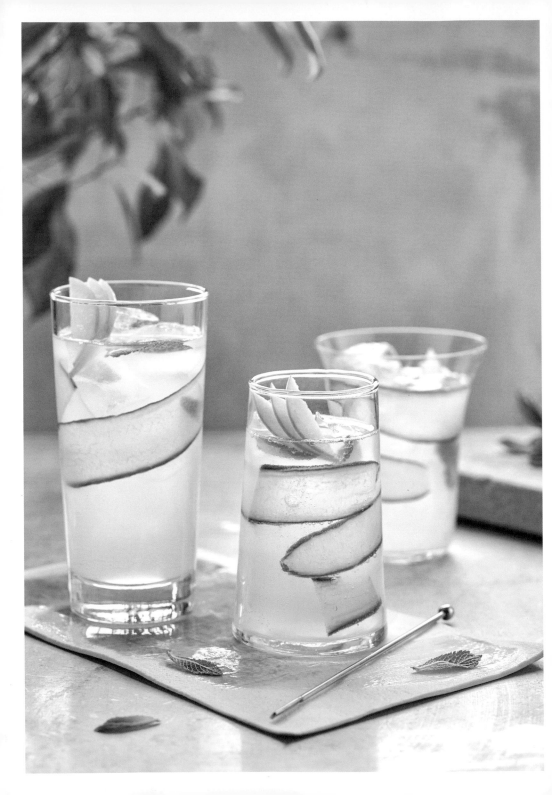

# Croquet

I've often wondered how cocktails get their names. The answer may well be simply because they perfectly evoke a mood, a period or a time of year – in this case, a summer afternoon playing croquet, or, for that matter, tennis. I've made it as an individual cocktail but it can easily be scaled up for a bigger group. As you'll be sober, of course, there will be no excuse for cheating. (Croquet can be a vicious game.)

**SERVES 1**

50ml (2fl oz) Seedlip Garden 108 or Ceder's Crisp alcohol-free spirit
50ml (2fl oz) chilled, unsweetened cloudy apple juice
100ml (3½fl oz) chilled cucumber tonic water
3–4 ice cubes
cucumber and apple slices and a sprig of mint, to garnish

Pour the alcohol-free spirit, apple juice and tonic water into a highball glass. Add the ice and stir.

Garnish with the slices of cucumber and apple and sprig of mint and serve.

Tip: If you want to make it really fancy, take a long, fine slice from a small cucumber and wrap it around the inside of the glass, as in the picture.

# Classic Virgin Mary

A Virgin Mary, the vodka-less version of a Bloody Mary, is one of the most iconic of alcohol-free cocktails, losing very little of the character of the vodka-laced original. That said, there's plenty of dispute about what that character should be – as with steak tartare (with which it actually goes remarkably well, see page 197), everyone has their own way of making it. I, for example, am not mad about the inclusion of celery salt, which I always feel makes it taste rather musty, so prefer to use ordinary sea salt or even a pinch of onion salt. Whatever you choose, it's best to add any seasoning bit by bit and keep tasting until it's just as you like it. I also think a Virgin Mary needs slightly more Worcestershire sauce than the alcoholic version does.

The great thing about this cocktail is that a 150ml (5fl oz) portion of tomato juice counts as one of your five a day, though be sure to get the best that you can lay your hands on. *Pictured on page 87.*

SERVES 1

150ml (5fl oz) tomato juice
5ml (1 teaspoon) freshly
  squeezed lemon juice
2 shakes of Tabasco sauce
3–4 shakes of
  Worcestershire sauce
  (see Tip)
pinch of celery salt, sea salt
  or onion salt
freshly ground black pepper
ice cubes
celery stick, to garnish

Pour the tomato juice and lemon juice into a jug and season with the Tabasco, Worcestershire sauce, salt and pepper. Give the mixture a good stir, then taste and adjust the seasoning.

Fill a tumbler with ice, pour over the Virgin Mary, add a celery stick to garnish and serve.

Tip: If you're vegetarian or vegan, make sure to use a suitable replacement for the Worcestershire sauce, as it usually contains anchovies.

# Smoky Mary

Here I've ramped up the smoky character of the drink by using chipotle sauce rather than a standard hot sauce and smoked salt or smoked water. *Pictured on page 87.*

SERVES 1

150ml (5fl oz) tomato juice
5–10ml (1–2 teaspoons) freshly squeezed lime juice
½–1 teaspoon chipotle hot sauce
2 shakes of Worcestershire sauce (use a vegan product if you're vegetarian or vegan)
pinch of smoked salt or a shake of smoked water and a pinch of ordinary sea salt
ice cubes

Pour the tomato juice and lime juice into a jug and season with the chipotle sauce, Worcestershire sauce and smoked salt, or smoked water and salt.

Give the mixture a good stir, then taste and adjust the seasoning.

Fill a tumbler with ice, pour over the Smoky Mary and serve.

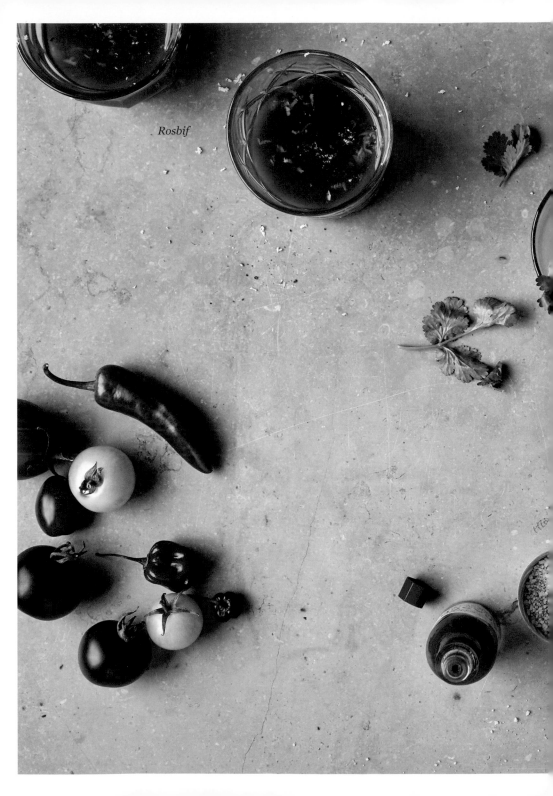

*Rosbif*

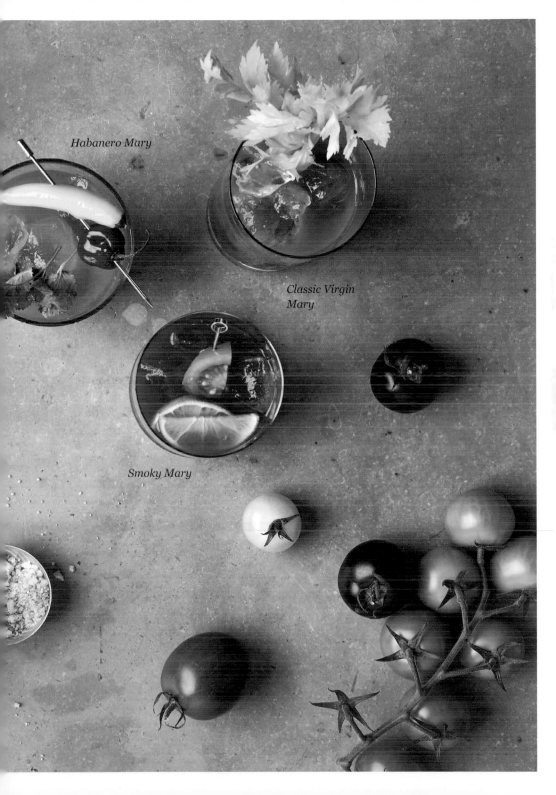

Habanero Mary

Classic Virgin
Mary

Smoky Mary

# Habanero Mary

If you can find yellow tomato juice for this extra-fiery version, do use it – the Isle of Wight growers The Tomato Stall make a delicious one. Or you could try making your own by blending and then straining some ripe yellow tomatoes. *Pictured on page 87.*

**SERVES 1**

150ml (5fl oz) yellow tomato juice
15ml (1 tablespoon) freshly squeezed lime juice
a few drops (or a shake) of habanero or Scotch bonnet sauce
pinch of sea salt
ice cubes
sprig of coriander or slice of lime, to garnish

Pour the tomato juice and lime juice into a jug and season with the habanero or Scotch bonnet sauce and sea salt. Give the mixture a good stir, then taste and adjust the seasoning.

Fill a tumbler with ice, pour over the Habanero Mary, garnish with a sprig of coriander or slice of lime and serve.

# Rosbif

A rather meaty take on a Virgin Mary, which it seemed somewhat discourteous to call a Beefy Mary, so I named it Rosbif because it reminds me of a roast dinner. Note that you need to get ahead with this one by infusing your alt-gin. Personally, I think this version is better without ice, but obviously feel free to add it, if you prefer. *Pictured on page 86.*

**SERVES 3**

100ml (3½fl oz) alcohol-free gin alternative
15g (½oz) peeled fresh horseradish root, finely grated, plus extra (optional) to serve
200ml (7fl oz) tomato juice
75ml (5 tablespoons) cold double-strength beef stock (use a beef stock cube or stockpot made up with half the recommended quantity of water)
a generous few shakes of Worcestershire sauce
a generous few grinds of black pepper
a few drops of white wine vinegar (optional)

Pour the alcohol-free gin alternative into a measuring jug and stir in the grated horseradish. Cover with a clean tea towel and leave to infuse overnight in the refrigerator.

Strain the alt gin through a fine sieve into a separate jug. Stir in the tomato juice and beef stock. Season generously with Worcestershire sauce and pepper, along with the vinegar if you think it needs it (I do).

Divide between three tumblers and grate over a little more fresh horseradish for those who want it (I'm up for that, too).

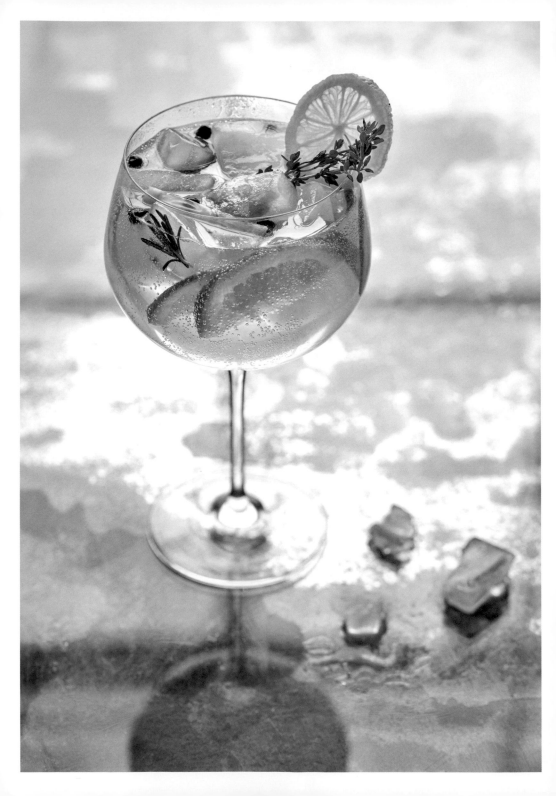

# NG&T

Although I love a G&T, I'm convinced that many of the things that make it so appealing – the tonic, the ice, the garnish, the glass – can be replicated in an alcohol-free drink. So much of a drink is about presentation. My local tapas bar, Bar 44, has recognized that and serves an alcohol-free G&T, which I quite often order when I'm in there. It comes in one of those huge goldfish-bowl-sized glasses with loads of orange and lemon slices and a few juniper berries floating around in it, which makes you feel like you're having a proper drink. Here's my slightly tweaked version. (The "N" obviously stands for "not".)

**SERVES 1**

4–5 ice cubes
2 slices each of orange and
    lemon
2–3 juniper berries
75ml (5 tablespoons)
    Juniper Syrup (see below)
tonic water (I like Fever-Tree
    Naturally Light), to top up

**FOR THE JUNIPER SYRUP
(MAKES 450ML/16FL OZ)**
400g (14oz) granulated or
    caster sugar
475ml (17fl oz) water
15 juniper berries, lightly
    crushed
finely pared rind of 1
    unwaxed lemon
finely pared rind of 1
    unwaxed lime

To make the juniper syrup, put the sugar in a saucepan and add the measured water. Heat over a low heat, stirring occasionally, until the sugar has completely dissolved. Add the juniper berries and citrus rinds and bring up to just below boiling point, then simmer for 10 minutes. Take off the heat and leave to cool.

Strain the syrup through a fine sieve into a wide-necked jug or bowl. Pour through a funnel into a sterilized bottle or jar, seal and store in the refrigerator for up to 2 weeks.

To make the NG&T, add the ice to a large glass, followed by the slices of orange and lemon and juniper berries, then pour in the juniper syrup. Top up with tonic water and serve.

**Tip:** You can buy juniper-flavoured spirit substitutes online instead of making juniper syrup, if you prefer.

# Chocolate Espresso Martini

One of the great things about the number of alcohol-free drinks on the market now is how easy it is to find a good base for a cocktail. The London-based company Tipplesworth is an example – I especially love their Espresso Martini mix, which can be shaken up just as well with an alcohol-free spirit as it can with vodka, though you may need to adjust the sweetness by adding an extra shot (or two) of espresso.

SERVES 2

double shot of espresso
2 teaspoons cocoa powder
ice cubes
100ml (4fl oz) alcohol-free
   spirit, such as Stryyk Not
   Vodka or Seedlip Spice 94
100ml (4fl oz) Espresso
   Martini cocktail mixer, such
   as Tipplesworth
2–4 roasted coffee beans, to
   garnish

Brew the espresso. Spoon the cocoa powder into a cocktail shaker, then pour over the espresso and leave to cool.

Once cool, add some ice to the cocktail shaker, along with the alcohol-free spirit and Espresso Martini mixer, and shake well.

Strain into two martini glasses and garnish each with a roasted coffee bean or two.

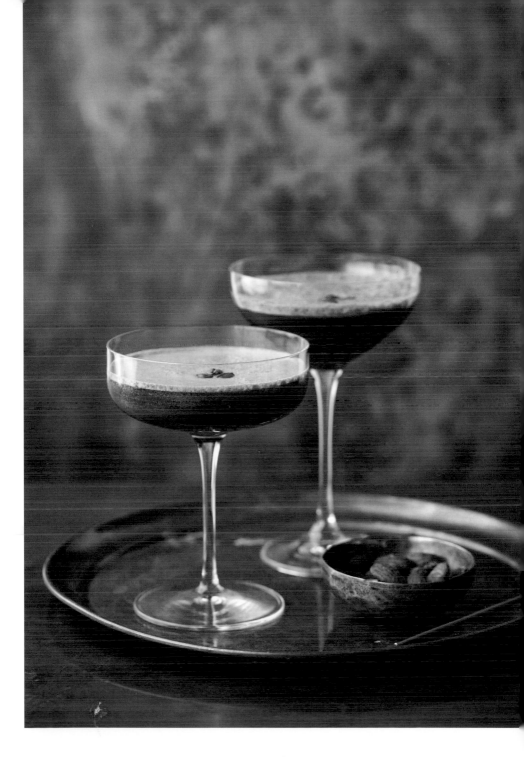

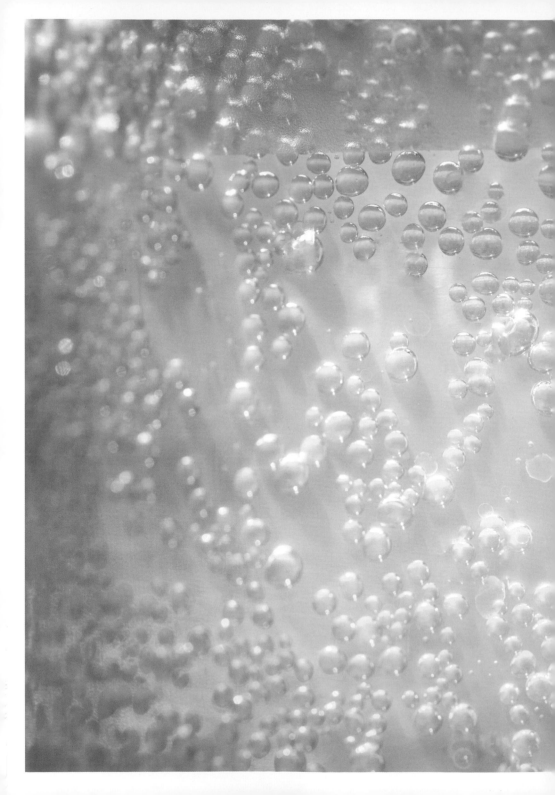

# ALCOHOL-FREE WINE, BEER AND CIDER-BASED DRINKS

Now that alcohol-free equivalents to beer and cider are so ubiquitous, you can use them to make almost any drink you would make with their full-strength equivalents. And alcohol-free wine – which is not quite there yet – is much improved by tweaking it with other ingredients, as you do with a Mulled "Wine" (see page 99), a sangria (see page 105) or – and this may be best of all – a Frosé (frozen rosé, see page 106).

So far as beer is concerned, you've still got the malt and the hops to play with. The simplest beer cocktail is a shandy (which you can actually make without any beer at all – see page 70 for my delicious lemonade and ginger beer version) or try a low-alcohol lager in the fiery Mexican beer cocktail, Michelada (see page 106).

You may have come across espresso stout, but there's no reason why you shouldn't add a dash of espresso to your alcohol-free stout if you're a coffee fiend (and if the stout doesn't already taste too strongly of coffee). Or an espresso martini mix, come to that.

With cider, sweetness can be an issue, less so if your base cider is made with traditional cider apples. You can always add a small splash of cider vinegar to make it more authentically "cidery". My favourite way of serving cider is to mull it (see page 99), but for a summer drink, you could make the equivalent of a fruit cider by adding a splash of fresh fruit cordial, a shrub or a few drops of fruit vinegar. (Don't be afraid, as I've already stressed, to play around with your drinks, just as you might experiment with different amounts of milk and sugar in your coffee.)

Wine, I admit, is trickier. Alcohol-free sparkling wine doesn't really cut it in cocktails in comparison to Champagne or even prosecco. Again, employ your own cordials – try the Rhubarb Cordial (see page 39) topped up with alcohol-free fizz for a delicious Bellini, or pour your fizz over a small scoop of sorbet, adding a dash of chilled soda water, to taste.

As far as still wines are concerned, you're better off making a white or red sangria (see page 105) or adapting one of those old recipes for white wine cups you find in vintage cookery books. (Truth be told, wine was probably rougher in those days than alcohol-free wines are now, which is why they added brandy to them. Obviously, that's not an option here, but you may want to chuck in an alcohol-free spirit for extra complexity and strength.)

Ambrose Heath's book *Good Drinks*, originally published in 1939, is an excellent source of inspiration and a good read, too. Also look for books on the art of entertaining by authors such as Elizabeth Craig and Countess Morphy, though you may have to disregard their predilection for orange squash.

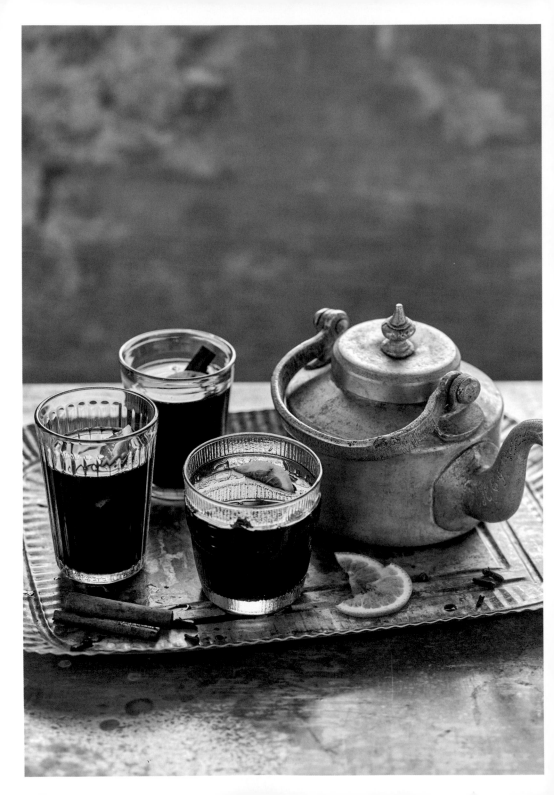

# Mulled "Wine"

I'm not convinced, as I've already mentioned, about alcohol-free wine – if you're a wine drinker, it really doesn't cut the mustard, but it does make a decent mulled wine, so much so that I found myself thinking when I first made this that I shouldn't really have a glass before I went out to dinner, before I remembered it was alcohol-free. The key is to add elderberry juice to give the drink body, but it is quite bitter, so you do need to add sugar (I like brown sugar) to taste.

SERVES 6–8

8 cloves
2 unwaxed oranges
75cl bottle alcohol-free red
    wine (I used Rawson's
    Retreat Cabernet
    Sauvignon)
330ml (11fl oz) elderberry
    juice (Biona is a good
    brand)
125g (4½oz) soft brown
    sugar
cinnamon stick
orange oil or orange bitters
    (optional)

Stick the cloves into the rind of one orange. Pour the alcohol-free wine and elderberry juice into a small–medium saucepan (you want the liquid to cover the orange), add 125g (4½oz) sugar, the cinnamon stick and 2–3 drops of orange oil or a shake of orange bitters and bring slowly up to simmering point over a low heat without letting it boil. Take off the heat and leave for 30 minutes to infuse.

To serve, reheat the mulled "wine". Slice the remaining orange and place a slice into six to eight small cups or heatproof glasses. Pour over the hot mulled "wine" and serve.

# Red Wine Hot Chocolate

If you have any Mulled "Wine" (see page 99) left over, you can use it to make Red Wine Hot Chocolate, a drink that took the internet by storm a couple of years ago. Or you can make it from scratch from alcohol-free red wine or elderberry juice. Feel free to play around with the quantities, depending on how intense and bitter you like your hot chocolate (I err on the dark side). The wine element may sound weird, but it adds a gorgeous berry fruitiness to the drink.

SERVES 2

1 tablespoon cocoa powder
¼ teaspoon ground
  cinnamon (unless you are
  using Mulled "Wine", see
  below)
200ml (7fl oz) whole milk
75ml (5 tablespoons)
  alcohol-free red wine or
  elderberry juice (or Mulled
  "Wine", see page 99)
1–2 squares of dark
  chocolate, plus a little
  grated, to garnish
squirty cream and/or
  marshmallows, to garnish

Put the cocoa powder and cinnamon (if using) in a small bowl. Heat the milk in a small saucepan over a medium heat until just below boiling, and pour enough over the cocoa to make a smooth, runny paste.

Pour the paste back into the saucepan with the rest of the milk. Add the "wine" and heat back to just below simmering point. Take off the heat, add the dark chocolate and stir until melted. Pour into two small mugs or heatproof glasses and top each with a generous squirt of cream and/or a couple of marshmallows. Finish with a grating of dark chocolate.

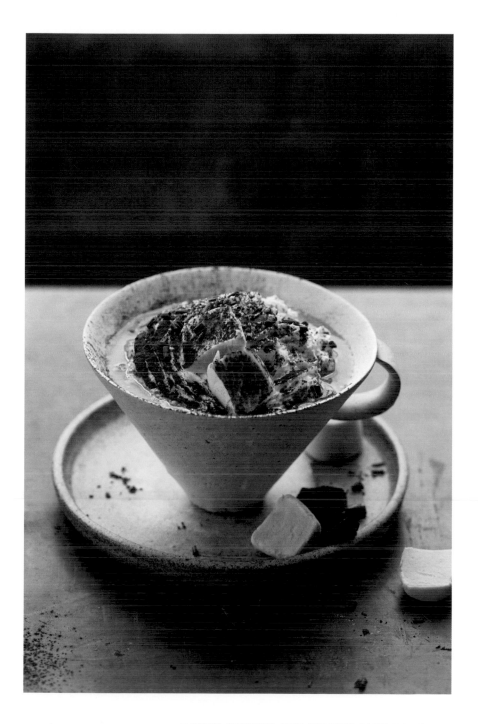

# Mulled "Cider" with Roasted Apples

Although you can mull apple juice on its own, I think it gives it an extra edge to use an alcohol-free cider and a dash of cider vinegar for sharpness. This is a really good drink to serve for Halloween or Bonfire Night, or for a Wassail party in early January (an old English custom which involves loudly beating pots and pans around the apple tree to scare off evil spirits and promote a good harvest).

SERVES 12–14

1 litre (1¾ pints) alcohol-free cider
2 tablespoons raw apple cider vinegar
1.5 litres (2¾ pints) unsweetened cloudy apple juice
2 thinly pared strips of unwaxed lemon rind
2 cinnamon sticks
8 cloves

FOR THE ROASTED APPLES
10–12 small Cox's apples or other small eating apples
about 50g (1¾oz) light muscovado sugar
100ml (3½fl oz) alcohol-free cider

To prepare the roasted apples, preheat the oven to 190°C/375°F/Gas Mark 5. Wash and core the apples, then score them around the middle. Put them in a baking dish and stuff the centre of each with the sugar – it's easiest to do this using the handle of a spoon or fork. Splash over the cider and roast for 45–50 minutes until soft and beginning to split.

Meanwhile, pour the main quantity of alcohol-free cider, vinegar and apple juice into a large saucepan and add the lemon rind, cinnamon sticks and cloves. Bring slowly up to simmering point over a low heat, then leave over a very low heat, without letting it boil, for about 30 minutes.

When the apples are ready, add them and their juices to the cider mixture. Taste, adding a little extra sugar if you think it needs it. Serve straight from the pan into heatproof glasses or cups, or transfer to a warmed bowl for serving.

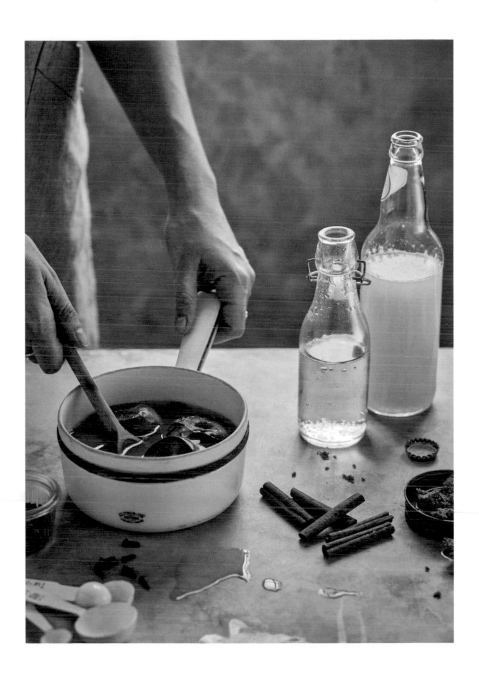

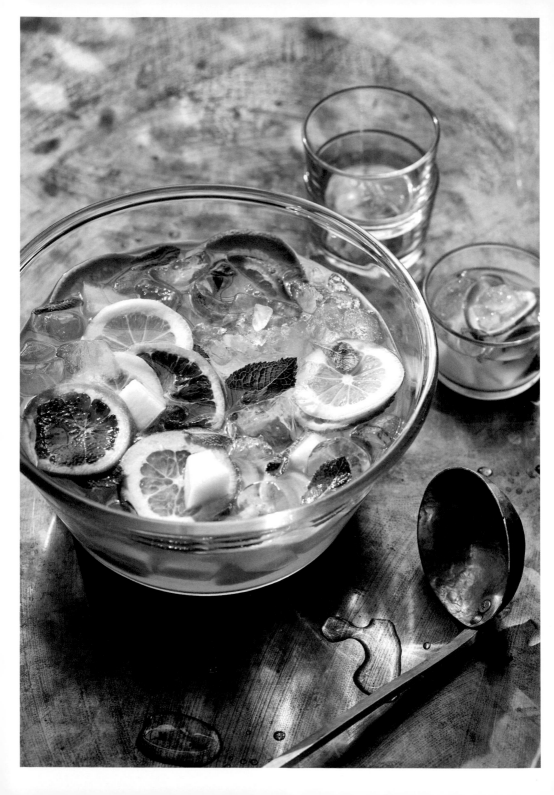

# White Sangria

Less well known but just as refreshing as its red counterpart, this absolutely looks and tastes the part on a hot summer's day. It's really worth including the melon and macerating it and the orange and lemon slices beforehand, as it gives the drink a lovely rounded sweetness.

**SERVES 4**

400ml (14fl oz) chilled alcohol-free Chardonnay-style white wine
25ml (scant 1fl oz) elderflower cordial
50ml (2fl oz) passion fruit syrup or cordial
wedge of honeydew or other ripe melon, peeled, deseeded and sliced
1 orange, sliced
1 lemon, sliced
2 dashes of Angostura bitters, or to taste
generous handful of ice cubes
chilled soda water, to top up
2 sprigs of mint, to garnish

Put the alcohol-free wine and cordials in a jug or bowl with the sliced fruit, and chill in the refrigerator for 45 minutes or so.

Stir the chilled sangria and add the Angostura bitters, then pour into a serving jug or bowl with the ice. Top up with soda water, garnish with the sprigs of mint and serve.

## VARIATION: TO MAKE RED SANGRIA

*Sangria recipes vary, but most contain some element of orange. I prefer using a dash of orange oil or an alcohol-free triple sec to orange juice, which will make the sangria cloudy. Macerate the fruit (oranges, lemons and maybe cherries or sliced nectarines in season) and "wine" (an alcohol-free Tempranillo is a good option) with some cinnamon-infused sugar syrup, then top up with lemonade or soda water.*

# Frosé

Frosé – frozen rosé – was a craze a couple of years ago, but you can equally well make it with an alcohol-free rosé "wine".

SERVES 2

225ml (8fl oz) alcohol-free
    rosé
110g (4oz) chilled ripe
    strawberries, hulled and
    sliced, plus 1 to garnish
2 tablespoons caster sugar
dash of grenadine or
    Hibiscus Syrup (see page
    170), optional

Pour the rosé into a plastic tub and freeze for 5–6 hours, forking it through every couple of hours.

Put the sliced strawberries in a bowl, sprinkle with the sugar and mix well. Leave to macerate in the refrigerator for 10–15 minutes, then stir and transfer to a blender. Add the frozen rosé and blend to a deep pink slush. Check for sweetness – add a dash of grenadine or hibiscus syrup to sweeten, if needed. Pour into two chilled glasses and garnish each with a slice of strawberry.

# Michelada

A Michelada is basically a Bloody Mary made with lager – or, in this case, alcohol-free lager. You can leave the clamato or other tomato juice out if you prefer, making it more of a chilli-and-lime-infused drink, but I like it.

SERVES 2

2–3 limes
chilli salt
ice cubes
100ml (3½fl oz) clamato, V8
    or tomato juice
Mexican or other hot sauce
    (I use a Chipotle sauce)
Worcestershire sauce
    (or vegetarian/vegan
    alternative)
330ml alcohol-free lager

Squeeze enough limes to give you 3–4 tablespoons of juice. Rub half a lime around the rims of two glasses. Dip the rims of the glasses into some chilli salt.

Put 3–4 ice cubes in each glass and pour over half the squeezed lime juice, the clamato, V8 or tomato juice, a good shake of hot sauce and a few drops of Worcestershire sauce and stir. Top up each glass with the alcohol-free lager, squeeze over some more lime juice and drop a lime wedge into each glass.

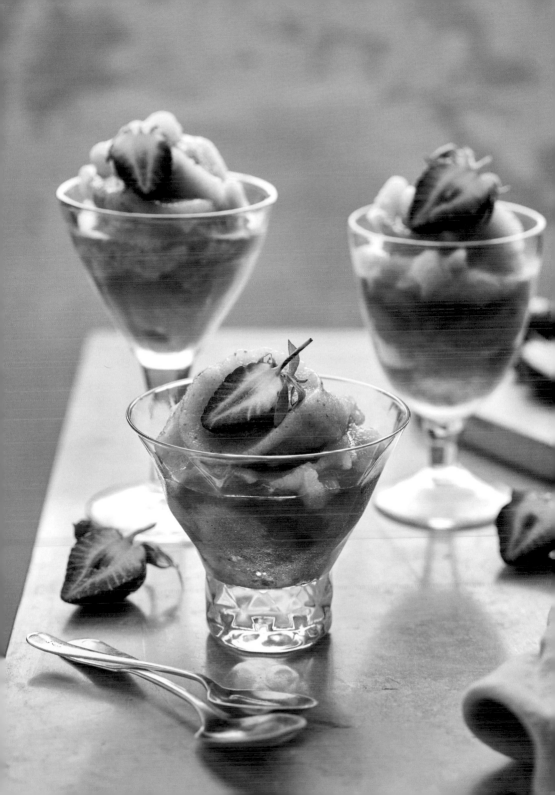

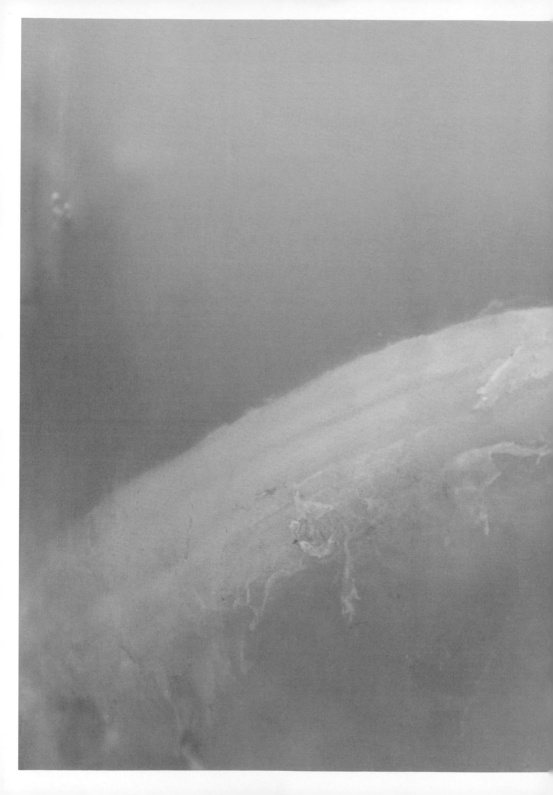

# FERMENTED DRINKS

Fermentation is the process that turns sugar into alcohol, so bear in mind that the following drinks could contain up to 2% ABV – not a problem for those who are cutting down, but it probably rules them out for those who are, for medical or other reasons, trying to avoid alcohol altogether.

They are in many ways the most exciting recipes in the book, but also the most time-consuming and complicated. If you think in terms of cooking, it's akin to making your own sourdough bread or yogurt, something you might well enjoy but equally well feel that life is too short and that you'd be better off buying a ready-made version.

With kombucha and kefir, which have become quite widely available, that is certainly an option and one I think I'd probably recommend for kombucha, unless you live somewhere without easy access to large supermarkets or health food shops. As I explain in the recipe on page 116, I was given the confidence to try it by a neighbour Caroline Gilmartin who runs fermentation classes and gave me a SCOBY (see the recipe for an explanation) to start me off. She also happens to be a biochemist and runs courses in Bristol, UK, for those of you who are of a similarly nervous disposition – you can find them on Eventbrite. There are bound to be similar ones in other cities. Obviously the bonus is that the kombuchas you make will be cheaper and fresher-tasting than the shop-bought versions.

Kefir, too, is worth making I think – and easier, as I explain, than making yogurt as you don't have to fiddle around getting your milk to the right temperature. I really like water kefir, too, especially when it's flavoured with other ingredients (see page 114). The combination with orange juice is particularly delicious.

Once you're on a roll with it, it's easy to keep up and incredibly good for your overall gut health, something that is outside the scope of this book, but which you may want to look into more closely online.

The two other drinks in this section are more obscure and therefore less easy to find elsewhere – at the time of writing, at least. Things change so fast these days we could find tepache, a Mexican fermented pineapple drink made from pineapple peel, on every street food stall in twelve months' time, especially given the popularity of tacos, with which it goes very well. Both it and kvass – a fermented rye bread drink from Eastern Europe made from dried rye bread crusts – are truly the drink world's equivalent of *cucina povera,* but punch well above their humble origins in taste terms with a flavour that's more akin to a beer. The kvass is really toasty.

If you're an adventurous cook who loves culinary experiments, I would definitely give them a try.

# Milk Kefir

The simplest ferment to start with is milk kefir, a cultured fermented drink that originates from central Asia. It's easiest to think of it like a supercharged yogurt, containing many more good bacteria – about 30 – compared to the 2–4 types in the average live yogurt, and therefore a much more powerful probiotic.

The beauty with making milk kefir is that you don't have to faff around with thermometers and you can use milk straight from the refrigerator, although the whole process will work faster if you start at room temperature.

The main issue is getting hold of kefir grains, which look less like grains than a little clump of milk solids – a bit like a small cauliflower floret. The ideal is to get your grains from someone who's already regularly making their own kefir. If you're starting from scratch with new grains, you'll need to begin with a smaller quantity of milk than in the recipe here, about 100ml (3½fl oz), and it may take longer for the thickening process to get underway. You can use dairy-free milk, but results are more reliable if you use whole cows' milk.

This makes enough for one or two people and about as much kefir as I can fit in the refrigerator along with everything else. If you want to make kefir for the whole family, simply double or treble the quantities, but while you're learning, I'd start small. Depending on how thick your kefir is, you can either drink it on its own or as a shake or a lassi, or dollop it over muesli.

**MAKES 375ML (13FL OZ)**

½ teaspoon (a small lump)
kefir grains (see recipe
introduction)
375ml (13fl oz) organic
cows' milk

Spoon the kefir grains into a sterilized 500-ml (18-fl oz) preserving jar and pour over the milk, leaving 2cm (¾ inch) of head space at the top. Close the jar and leave on a work surface or shelf at room temperature for 18–24 hours, depending on how warm the room is, or until the kefir has thickened slightly but is still a drinkable consistency. The longer you ferment kefir, the thicker – and tangier – it will get.

Carefully fish out the starter grains and set them aside to make the next batch. Pour the milk kefir through a funnel into a sterilized bottle or other airtight container, seal and store in the refrigerator for up to 4–5 days.

Start your next batch of kefir in the same way, reusing your starter grains. If making a fresh batch at a later date, store the starter grains covered with a little fresh milk in an airtight container in the refrigerator for up to 6 weeks or in the freezer.

*VARIATION: FLAVOURED KEFIR*

*If you prefer your milk kefir flavoured, divide the kefir up between smaller bottles and add a flavouring ingredient. My favourite by far is a finely pared strip or two of unwaxed lemon rind, but you could add other citrus rind, like orange or grapefruit, if that appeals to you more. Bear in mind that kefir is slightly tart, so flavourings such as vanilla or cocoa aren't going to work unless you also add Sugar Syrup (see page 14).*

# Water Kefir

Water kefir is similar to milk kefir but uses a different type of grain. They work in much the same way except you need more of them and they take longer to ferment. You end up with a cloudy, slightly sweet liquid that you can use to dilute juices or cordials, or flavour as you choose (see below).

**MAKES 800ML (1⅔ PINTS)**

30g (1oz) granulated or
   caster sugar
100ml (3½fl oz) boiling
   water
700ml (1¼ pints) cold water
30g (1oz) water kefir grains

Put the sugar in a bowl, pour over the boiling water and stir until the sugar has completely dissolved. Top up with the measured cold water and leave to cool.

Spoon the grains into a sterilized 1-litre (1¾-pint) preserving jar and pour over the cooled sugar solution and remaining water, leaving about 3cm (1¼ inches) of head space at the top. Loosely seal the jar and leave on a work surface at room temperature for about 3 days or until the liquid turns cloudy and no longer tastes sweet.

Strain the liquid through a fine sieve into a wide-mouthed jug and reserve the grains for the next batch. Either pour the water kefir through a funnel into a sterilized bottle or other airtight container, seal and store in the refrigerator for up to 4–5 days, or flavour it as suggested.

---

*FLAVOURED WATER KEFIRS*
*Water kefir is more versatile than milk kefir, as it lends itself to a wider variety of flavours. Try adding the following ingredients to a 250ml (9fl oz) bottle of water kefir and leave it to ferment in the refrigerator for another 24 hours – it will get slightly fizzy, so open with care!*
- *A sprig of rosemary (my favourite way to flavour water kefir)*
- *2 slices of fresh root ginger*
- *A sliver of unwaxed lemon rind*

### VARIATION 1: ORANGE KEFIR WATER
Simply mix 100ml (3½fl oz) freshly squeezed orange juice with an equal amount of water kefir and a dash of orange flower water, and serve.

### VARIATION 2: COCONUT KEFIR
Follow the recipe for water kefir but use coconut water instead of ordinary water. If the coconut water is already sweetened, you should need less sugar than the standard recipe.

### VARIATION 3: PICKLED CUCUMBER KEFIR
This won't be for everyone – it's quite sour, but refreshing. Use the pickling liquid from a jar of Polish-style pickled cucumbers in sweet vinegar – I use 150ml (5fl oz) water kefir to 75ml (5 tablespoons) pickling liquid.

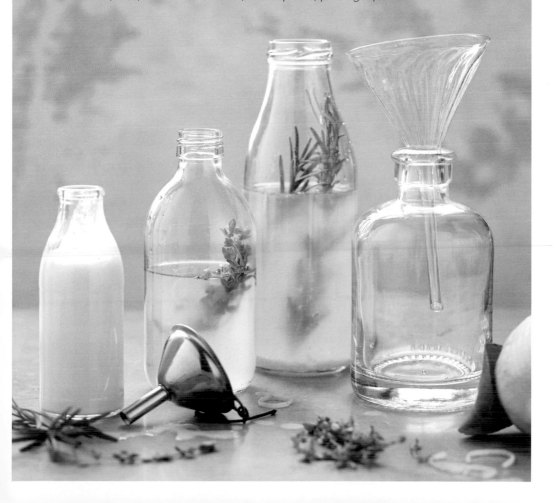

# Kombucha

Kombucha is a fermented tea-based drink, which I have to admit is more of an undertaking to make at home than kefir. It takes longer, about two weeks, and involves an unnerving ingredient called a SCOBY (an acronym for symbiotic culture of bacteria and yeast) – a slithery disc that looks as if it might have dropped in from outer space, which you can beg from a fellow kombucha brewer or buy online. Kombucha recipes are also habitually accompanied by warnings of the dire consequences of not maintaining scrupulous levels of hygiene – in fact, I was so unnerved I decided not to take mine along to a talk I was doing on alcohol-free drinks in case I killed off my audience.

Having alarmed you by saying all that, many people make kombucha with great success and have done so for several centuries, so don't let me put you off. It is a deliciously refreshing drink with more personality than a water kefir, and once you're on a roll with it, it's not that hard to do. It doesn't matter hugely which kind of tea you use, though to start with I'd advocate ordinary black tea. Given the amount of time it takes to make, you might want to double the recipe while you're about it.

*VARIATION: FLAVOURED KOMBUCHA*
*You can flavour your kombucha with raw ingredients like fresh root ginger or add fruit juice (I like pink grapefruit juice) to get it bubbling away. You may have already developed a taste for particular combinations from shop-bought kombucha, but personally I find lemon and ginger works really well, as do frozen berries such as blueberries and raspberries, which you don't need to defrost first.*

**MAKES 1 LITRE (1¾ PINTS)**

50g (1¾oz) granulated sugar
2 black tea bags or 2–3g
(1–1½ tablespoons) loose
black tea
800ml (28fl oz) boiling or
just off boiling water
200ml (7fl oz) kombucha
starter liquid, unflavoured
live kombucha or
kombucha from a previous
batch
1 disc of SCOBY (see recipe
introduction

Put the sugar and tea bags or tea leaves in a sterilized 1.2-litre (2-pint) glass jar, pour over the measured boiling or just off boiling water and stir. Leave to brew for 3 minutes. Remove the tea bags or strain off the tea leaves and leave to cool. Add the kombucha starter and SCOBY, then cover with a piece of muslin secured with a rubber band. Leave in a cool, dark place for about 5–7 days, checking it occasionally. Once it starts fermenting, you'll begin to see small bubbles forming on the surface and signs of new growth on the SCOBY itself. Taste the kombucha – it should be fresh and tart but not vinegary. If it's too sweet, leave it to ferment a bit longer.

Carefully remove and set aside the SCOBY, strain the kombucha through a fine sieve into a wide-necked jug, then pour through a funnel into sterilized smaller glass bottles, reserving some for making your next batch of kombucha, and leaving about 2cm (¾ inch) of head space at the top of the bottles before sealing. Alternatively, pour the kombucha into another sterilized jar or jars, add some fruit or other flavouring ingredients (see opposite) and cover as before. Return the bottles or jars to the cupboard and leave for a further 2–3 days until fizzy, then refrigerate before drinking. If you have flavoured the kombucha, strain off the flavouring ingredients and bottle it as with the unflavoured kombucha. It should keep in the refrigerator for 2–3 weeks.

Make another infusion of sweet tea as before and cool, then add the starter and SCOBY and get your next batch fermenting in the same way.

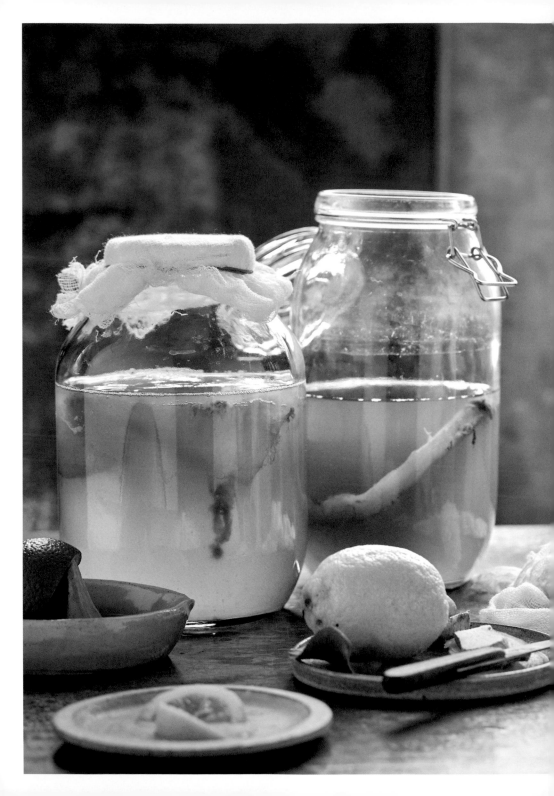

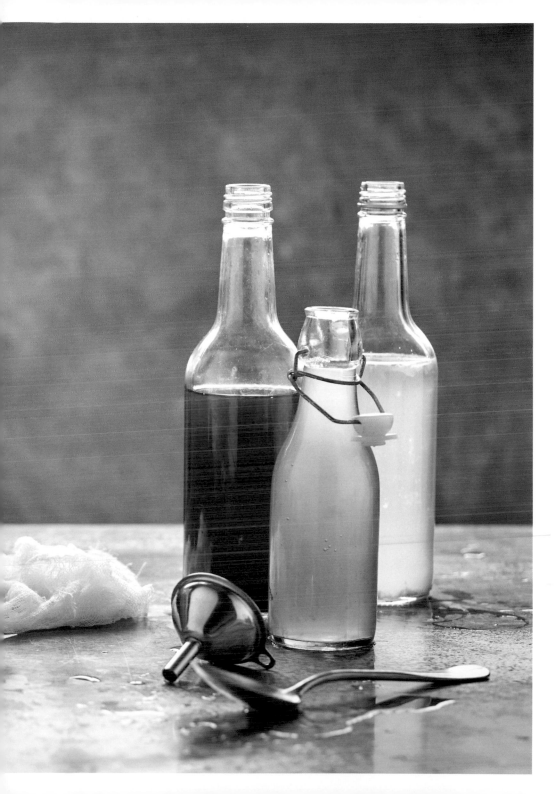

# Olia Hercules's Kvass

Fermenting dried bread crusts doesn't sound that appetizing, but kvass turned out to be one of my favourite drinks in the book. Like other ferments, it's refreshingly sour but surprisingly full flavoured – it tastes a bit like a toasty beer.

According to my friend Olia Hercules, author of the best-selling cookbook *Mamushka*, it has been made in Eastern Europe for over a thousand years. Alexander Pushkin wrote in *Yevgeny Onegin* that "they needed kvass as much as air", and kvass making was indeed as big as bread baking from antiquity to the commercial version sold from trucks in the Soviet Union.

Unlike many kvass recipes, Olia's version doesn't use commercial yeast – she adds a tablespoon of her rye sourdough starter to the jar and says it bubbles up on day two. Alternatively, you can use a tablespoon of organic rye flour, or rye bread on its own can kick off the fermentation process; it will just take longer. Here's Olia's recipe.

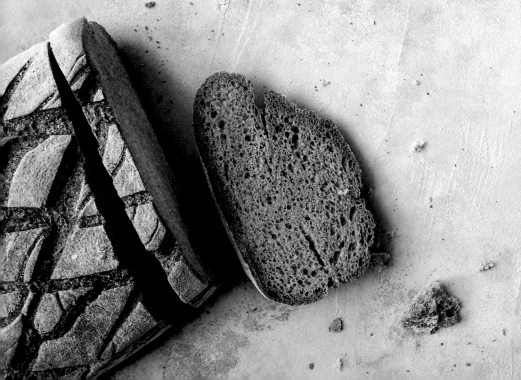

If your bread is fresh, leave it to go very
dry or dry it out in a low oven, then turn
the heat up for 5 minutes or so to accentuate
the toasty flavour. Put it together with all the remaining
ingredients in a sterilized 2.1-litre (3²/₃-pint) preserving
jar and seal. Leave somewhere warm for a few days
to ferment, checking every other day – I left mine for
4 days, but it could possibly have done with a little
longer. You can remove some of the bread and top it
up with fresh dried rye bread to speed the process up.

Strain the kvass through a colander into a wide-necked
jug, then strain through a muslin-lined funnel into
two sterilized 75cl glass bottles, seal and store in the
refrigerator for up to 5 days. Save some of the thicker
liquid at the bottom of each bottle to help kick start
the next batch.

### VARIATION: FLAVOURED KVASS

As with other fermented drinks, you can flavour
your kvass with herbs or fruits. Traditionally,
these would have been foraged from the
surrounding countryside, so fruit, such as wild
cherries, elderberries and blackberries, would
all work well, as would home-grown raspberries
and apples. There are some good suggestions
in the Russian Kitchen section of the Russia
Beyond website. You can also make kvass out of
beetroot without using bread, which is more like
a liquid pickle.

**MAKES ABOUT 1.5 LITRES
(2¾ PINTS)**

150g (5½oz) organic dark
  rye bread
1.7 litres (3 pints) water
1 tablespoon organic
  wholemeal rye flour or rye
  starter mixed with 30ml
  (2 tablespoons) water
4 tablespoons organic
  honey (or agave syrup)
  diluted with 60ml
  (4 tablespoons) warm
  water, for ease of mixing
handful of organic raisins
1 tablespoon coriander
  seeds, lightly toasted and
  crushed
1 tablespoon caraway
  seeds, lightly toasted and
  crushed

# Tepache

Tepache (pronounced *teh-patchay*) is a Mexican fermented pineapple drink that can be made from just the skin of the pineapple, but I think it tastes better and more fruity using at least some of the flesh, too. Piloncillo, which comes in solid cones, is the authentic sugar to use, available from Mexican grocery stores or online, but any brown sugar will do.

**MAKES ABOUT 750ML (1⅓ PINTS)**

125g (4½ oz) demerara or other brown sugar, preferably organic, or piloncillo (see recipe introduction)
500ml (18fl oz) filtered water
piece of cinnamon stick or bark
3–4 cloves
1 small–medium ripe sweet pineapple, preferably organic
ice cubes and soda water, to serve
slice of lime and/or sprig of mint, to garnish

Put the sugar in a saucepan and pour over the filtered water. Heat over a very low heat, stirring occasionally, until the sugar has completely dissolved. Add the cinnamon and cloves, then leave to cool.

Wash the pineapple, then cut off the top and base. Quarter, cutting away the hard central core, cut into chunks and bruise lightly with a meat mallet or rolling pin. Pack as much of the peel and chunks as you can into a sterilized 1.5-litre (2¾-pint) preserving jar. Pour over the cooled sugar solution and extra water if needed to ensure that the pineapple is submerged. Give the contents of the jar a stir, then scrunch a piece of nonstick baking paper into the top of the jar to keep the pineapple pieces submerged. Secure a piece of muslin over the top of the jar and leave for 2–3 days at room temperature, checking it regularly. Once you see the liquid starting to froth up, the fermentation has got going. Taste it and see how you like it at that stage, and if necessary leave it to ferment a bit longer (though not too long, otherwise it may acquire some alcohol in the process). Strain the liquid into a jug, then pour through a funnel into a sterilized 75cl glass bottle, seal and store in the refrigerator for up to 5 days.

Serve over ice with a splash of soda water, each garnished with a slice of lime and/or sprig of mint.

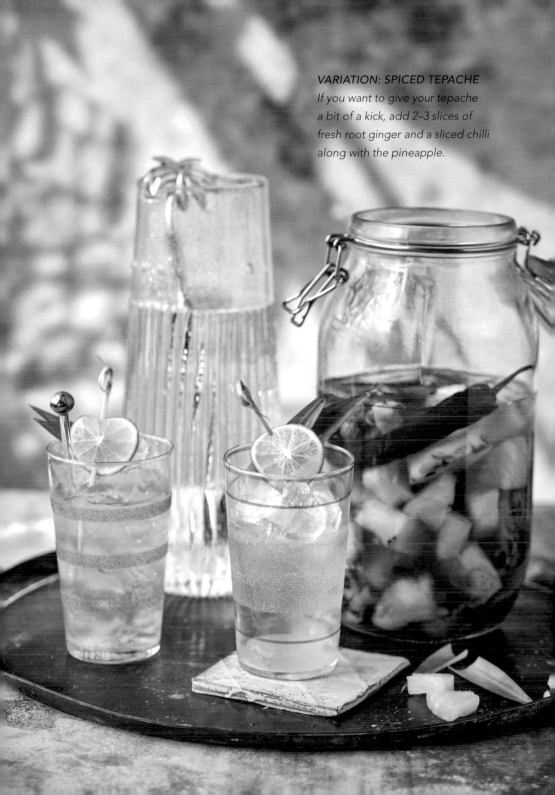

**VARIATION: SPICED TEPACHE**
*If you want to give your tepache
a bit of a kick, add 2–3 slices of
fresh root ginger and a sliced chilli
along with the pineapple.*

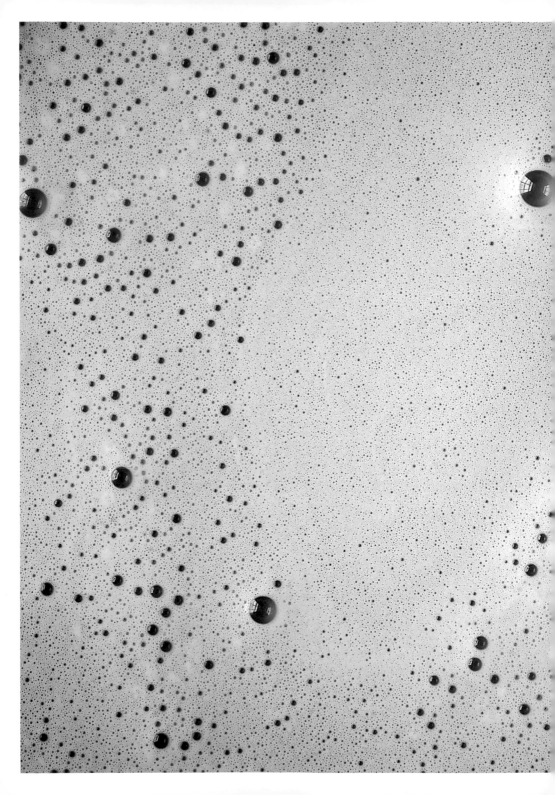

# LATTES, SHAKES AND LASSIS

One of the biggest changes in recent years in the products that are available to us to drink and cook with is the number of dairy-free milks that are now on the market. The quality has massively improved, with an incredible range of flavours: you can buy soy milk, oat milk, almond and various other nut milks, rice milk and coconut milk, to name a few. As the English firm Rude Health nicely put it "We now live in a world where there is a dairy alternative for everyone, tree huggers and milk chuggers alike."

Because it's fun to experiment with what's on the market, and there's a massive interest in vegan-friendly options, I've made most of these recipes with dairy-free milks, but you can equally well make them with cows' milk. In general, I find whole milk works better than semi-skimmed. I usually buy organic.

Although I'm personally committed to dairy (not least because I don't want to see farmers go out of business and the ensuing change to the countryside that would result), I do think some drinks taste better with a dairy-free alternative. That includes, for me, most lattes – dairy milk makes them over-rich and creamy to my mind, which dumbs down the other flavours in the drink, but you may well disagree. Milkshakes, on the other hand, or flavoured milk drinks like the Lavender Milk on page 138, are delicious with dairy milk, the creamier the better. Adding ice cream (essential in any milkshake, in my humble opinion) will also do that job. I have, however, given a dairy-free milkshake recipe for the vegans among you.

Yogurt is also a friend in the refrigerator if you're whipping up drinks – again, dairy-free versions are ubiquitous these days.

I must say I love a lassi with a curry. The Mango Lassi on page 142 is just ridiculously easy and if you're a cardamom fan (join the club), you'll love the Banana, Coconut and Cardamom Lassi on page 141, too. You'll find more in the Juices and Smoothies section (a smoothie, of course, being a lassi by another name). And if you're into making milk kefir, you can use that, too.

Some of you may worry about the calorie content of some of the drinks in this chapter, especially the shakes, but so long as you're not drinking them every day, I don't see the problem. Everyone deserves a treat, especially if they're not drinking. And even shakes, especially milkshakes, have nutritional value given that milk contains not only calcium and protein, but important vitamins and minerals, too.

# Turmeric Latte

Aka golden mylk, turmeric latte has been one of the iconic vegan drinks of the last couple of years, widely offered in cafés but actually quite simple to make at home. The whisking may sound like a bit of a performance, but it's actually key to the drink, integrating the spices and giving it a luxuriant foamy texture. You may find you need slightly more turmeric depending on the strength and freshness of the one you have, while the pepper helps to activate its health-giving properties.

**MAKES 1 MUG OR 2 SMALLER CUPS**

225ml (8fl oz) coconut, almond or oat milk (I particularly like Rebel Kitchen Mylk, which contains coconut cream, brown rice and cashew)
½ teaspoon ground turmeric
¼ teaspoon ground cinnamon
⅛ teaspoon ground ginger
⅛ teaspoon finely ground black pepper
1 teaspoon agave or maple syrup, or honey (if you're not vegan)

Pour the milk into a saucepan and add all the remaining ingredients. Heat over a moderate heat, whisking all the time with a small balloon whisk or milk frother.

Pour into the mug or cups, through a fine strainer if you want a smoother texture.

*VARIATION: CHAI*

*If you like the taste of turmeric latte you may also like chai, a sweet milky tea spiced with cardamom, cinnamon, nutmeg, cloves and other spices. You simply infuse the teabags and spices in the milk – with can be dairy or non-dairy – for about 10 minutes. You can also buy ready-made chai teabags.*

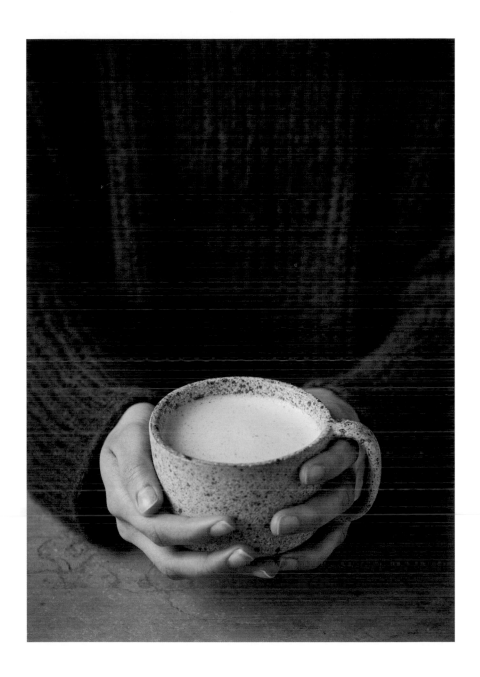

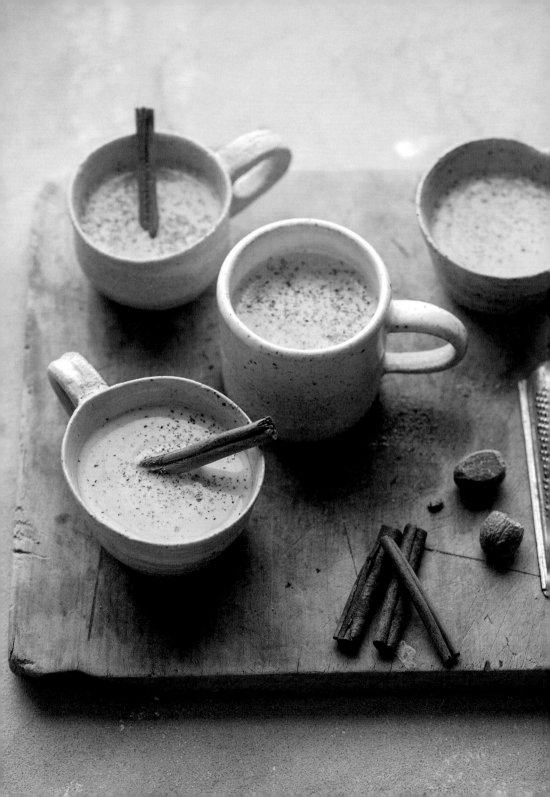

# Spiced Pumpkin Latte

A bit of a coffee shop classic, especially around Halloween and Thanksgiving, but to tell the truth, I prefer this without coffee. You could make the pumpkin purée yourself, but it actually tastes better canned. Do check whether or not it's sweetened, and if it is, you may need less maple syrup, though probably not if you've got a sweet tooth!

**SERVES 2**

2 tablespoons unsweetened pumpkin purée, about 40g (1½oz) in total
¼ teaspoon mixed spice or a pinch each of ground cinnamon, ginger and nutmeg
½ teaspoon vanilla extract
2 tablespoons maple syrup
200ml (7fl oz) oat or almond milk, or whole dairy milk if you're not vegan or dairy intolerant
ground cinnamon, to serve

Put the pumpkin purée and spice in a small saucepan and stir to mix. Add the vanilla extract and maple syrup, then mix in the milk. Heat over a moderate heat, whisking all the time with a small balloon whisk or milk frother, until just below boiling point.

Pour into two latte glasses or mugs and sprinkle over a little ground cinnamon to serve.

# Matcha Latte

If you've never really taken to green tea, give this delicious latte a go, only be careful not to scald the powder – that's what makes green tea bitter. You'll also need something to froth up your milk, but don't overdo it, otherwise you'll be left with a lot of green air. I like to make it in a bowl rather than a mug.

**SERVES 1**

½ teaspoon matcha tea powder, plus a little extra to serve
1 tablespoon water
1–2 teaspoons golden caster sugar or agave or maple syrup, or honey if you're not vegan (quantity depending on whether or not your milk is sweetened)
125ml (4fl oz) almond, rice or soy milk

Measure out the matcha into a bowl. Add the measured water and 1 teaspoon of whatever sweetener you're using and whisk together until you have a smooth paste. A traditional Japanese bamboo whisk is good for this, but a miniature balloon whisk is fine.

Pour the milk into a saucepan and heat over a low heat, whisking it up a bit but not over-whisking, until just below boiling point – if you can dip your finger in the mixture comfortably, it's probably the right temperature.

Whisk the milk into the matcha and check for sweetness, adding a little more sugar, syrup or honey to taste. Sift a little matcha powder on top to serve.

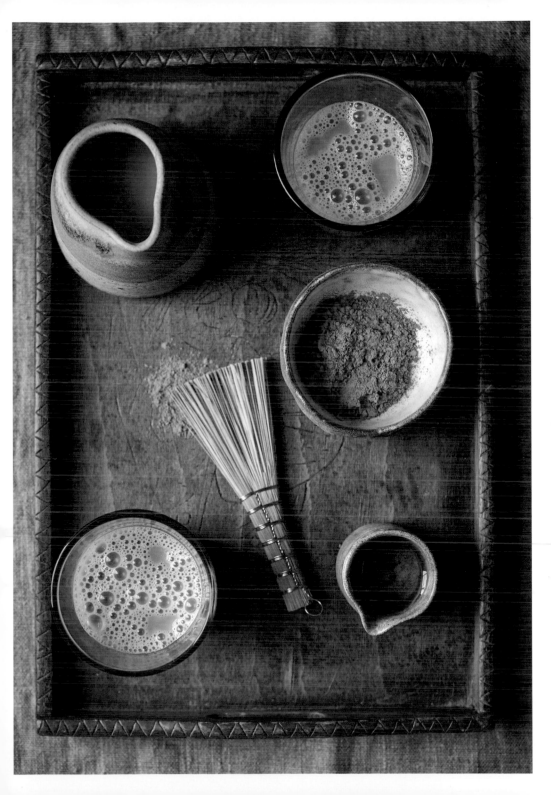

# Roasted Almond Milkshake

This was inspired by a Spanish and Mexican drink called *horchata*, an almond or other nut-flavoured milk drink. I find the Mexican version too sweet and the Spanish one, which is made from tiger nuts, too much trouble to make from scratch. So follow me and cheat with this easy version. For the finishing sprinkle, you can buy praline powder from specialist food suppliers or make your own – just melt 75g (2¾ oz) of granulated or caster sugar in a saucepan over a low–medium heat, then simmer without stirring until it turns a rich brown. Stir in a handful of whole, blanched almonds. Pour onto a nonstick baking tray, leave to cool and then blitz to a powder in a food processor. *Pictured on page 136.*

SERVES 2

2 scoops of dairy-free vanilla
  ice cream
250ml (9fl oz) chilled roasted
  almond milk or other nut
  milk, or whole dairy milk
dash of amaretto syrup or
  other almond-flavoured
  syrup, or more to taste if
  using dairy milk
small pinch of salt (optional,
  but it brings out the
  almond flavour)
praline powder, to serve
  (see recipe introduction)

Put all the ingredients (except the praline powder) in a blender and blend on high speed until the milkshake is smooth and frothy.

Divide between two glasses and sprinkle over some praline powder to serve.

# Super Strawberry Milkshake

Unless your strawberries are exceptionally ripe or you're using a strawberry ice cream, you generally need to boost the strawberry flavour here in some way with a strawberry syrup – or the Rhubarb Cordial on page 39, as rhubarb has a real affinity with strawberries. *Pictured on pages 136–7.*

SERVES 2

250g (9oz) ripe strawberries, plus extra to garnish (optional)
1 tablespoon caster sugar
2 scoops of dairy-free vanilla or strawberry ice cream, plus extra to serve (optional)
100ml (3½fl oz) unsweetened oat or other dairy-free milk
strawberry syrup or Rhubarb Cordial (see page 39), to taste (optional)
freeze-dried strawberry powder, to serve

Hull and slice the strawberries into a bowl, sprinkle with the sugar and mix well. Leave to macerate for 10 minutes.

Transfer to a blender and blend until smooth. Add the ice cream and milk and blend again. Taste and add a dash of strawberry syrup or rhubarb cordial to boost the strawberry flavour if necessary, then blend once more.

Pour into chilled glasses. If you like, serve with an extra scoop of ice cream, garnish with more strawberries, and sprinkle over a little freeze-dried strawberry powder to finish.

# Iced Coffee Shake

I never used to be that keen on iced coffee, but this coffee shake is another thing entirely. Why does ice cream make everything taste better? No need to answer that...

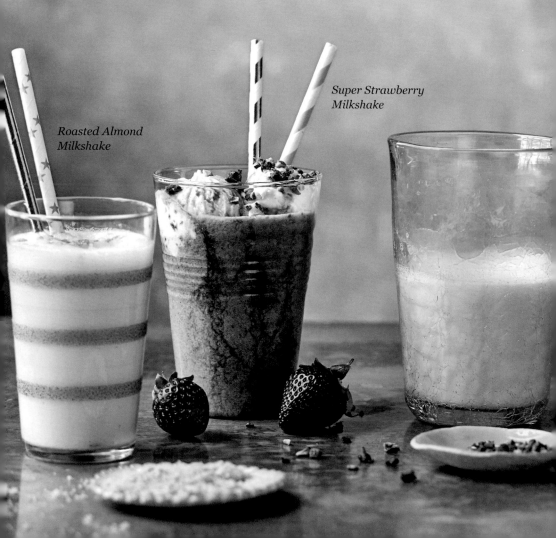

*Roasted Almond Milkshake*

*Super Strawberry Milkshake*

SERVES 1

50ml (2fl oz) Espresso
Martini cocktail mixer,
such as Tipplesworths or
2 shots of espresso and
2 teaspoons granulated
sugar
scoop of dairy-free or dairy
vanilla or coffee ice cream
100ml (3½fl oz)
unsweetened soy or other
dairy-free milk
dark chocolate for grating
or cocoa powder, to serve

If you're using coffee rather than an Espresso Martini
mixer, make it up, sweeten it and let it cool.

Add the Espresso Martini mixer or cooled sweetened
espresso to a blender with the ice cream and milk and
blend until frothy.

Pour into a highball glass and grate over a little dark
chocolate or sprinkle over a small pinch of cocoa
powder to serve.

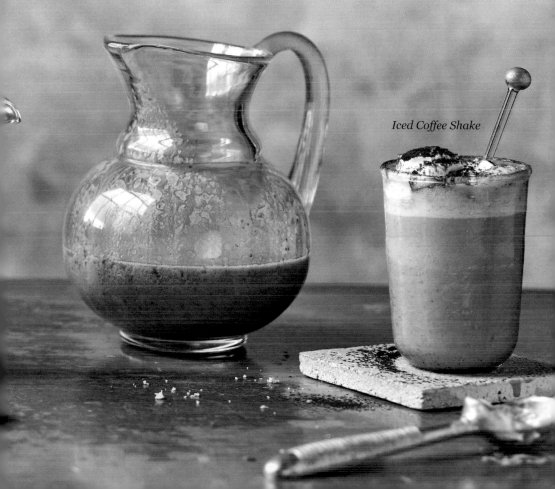

*Iced Coffee Shake*

# Lavender Milk

There's something wonderfully romantic about lavender, conjuring up visions of warm summer afternoons in an English country garden. So I loved the very idea of this lavender milk from mixologist Jack Adair Bevan, formerly of The Ethicurean at Wrington in Somerset, and was just smitten when I tasted it. It's just ridiculously good.

**SERVES 1**

ice cubes
30ml (2 tablespoons)
   lavender syrup (shop-
   bought or homemade
   – see below)
200ml (7fl oz) whole organic
   dairy milk or oat milk
lavender flower, to garnish

**FOR THE LAVENDER SYRUP**
   (MAKES 100ML/3½FL OZ)
100g (3½oz) granulated
   sugar
100ml (3½fl oz) water
10 heads of lavender, stalks
   removed

To make the lavender syrup, put the sugar in a saucepan and add the measured water. Heat over a low heat, stirring occasionally, until the sugar has completely dissolved. Bring to the boil, then add the lavender and simmer for a minute. Take off the heat, cover and leave to infuse for 40 minutes.

Strain the contents of the pan through a fine sieve into a wide-necked jug or bowl, then pour the liquid through a funnel into a sterilized bottle or other airtight container, seal and store in a cool place for up to 2 months. Once opened, store in the refrigerator for up to 2 weeks.

To make Lavender Milk, fill a glass with ice, then pour in the lavender syrup and milk and stir to mix, or for a more aerated drink, shake them together in a cocktail shaker. Garnish with a lavender flower.

*VARIATION: LAVENDER MILKSHAKE*
*Simply blend the lavender milk with a scoop of dairy or dairy-free vanilla ice cream, though you may want to up the syrup slightly.*

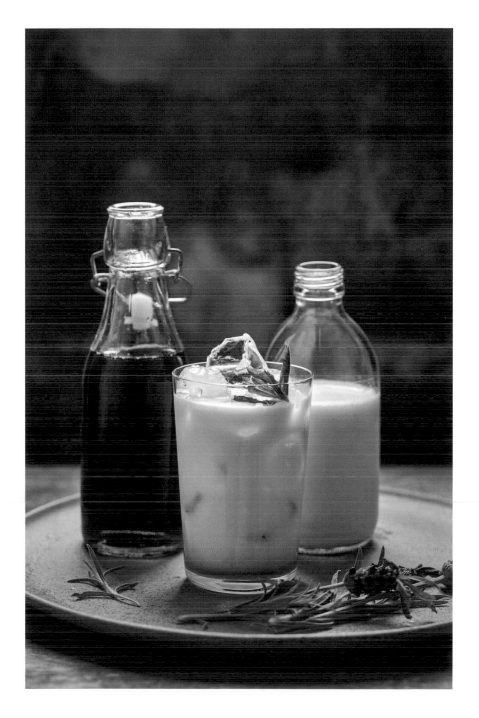

# Frozen Raspberry, Coconut and Chia Shake

Frozen raspberries are brilliant to have in the freezer because they can easily be whipped up into an instantly chilled smoothie or shake. They go beautifully with coconut, as this recipe proves. I've added chia seeds for added nutritional value (I mean, the coconut is a bit wicked), but you can choose not to.

SERVES 2

125g (4½ oz) frozen raspberries, straight from the freezer
300ml (10fl oz) coconut milk
1 tablespoon chia seeds (optional)
1–2 tablespoons Sugar Syrup (see page 14), optional
freeze-dried raspberries or raspberry powder, to serve (optional)

Put the frozen raspberries in a blender, pour in half the coconut milk and blend until smooth. Add the remaining coconut milk and the chia seeds, if using, and blend again. Check for sweetness – if you're using a sweetened coconut milk, you may not need extra sugar, but otherwise add the sugar syrup to taste.

Divide the shake between two glasses and sprinkle over some freeze-dried raspberries or raspberry powder, if you have some, to serve.

*VARIATION: FROZEN RASPBERRY, ALMOND AND CHIA SHAKE*
*Replace the coconut milk with almond milk and add a splash of orgeat or other almond syrup to taste.*

# Banana, Coconut and Cardamom Lassi

I wasn't sure whether to make this a smoothie or a lassi; it actually works as both. The lassi is slightly more savoury, while the smoothie is sweeter. Adjust the quantities depending on how banana-y, coconutty and cardamom-y you want it.

**SERVES 2**

1 medium-large ripe banana, preferably organic (wait until the skin has developed a few black spots)

2 heaped tablespoons dairy or dairy-free coconut yogurt

¼ teaspoon ground cardamom, or a little more to taste

100ml (3½fl oz) water

Peel and slice the banana into a blender or food processor. Add the coconut yogurt and ground cardamom and blend until smooth. Add the measured water and whizz again.

Divide between two glasses and serve.

**Tip:** To ice the lassi, put 3–4 ice cubes in the blender and crush before you add the other ingredients. Leave out the water.

> *VARIATION: BANANA, COCONUT AND CARDAMOM SMOOTHIE*
>
> *To turn this into a creamy smoothie, replace the water with 100ml coconut milk – or regular milk, depending on how strong the coconut flavour of your yogurt is – and add a teaspoon of honey or agave syrup before whizzing it up.*

# Mango Lassi

I almost always use canned mango pulp or purée for this (see page 12), as it's really hard to get mangoes that are ripe enough to blend, and if they are, they're almost impossible to peel. In the past, I always used yogurt to make lassi, but I now prefer the taste of milk kefir, which is slightly tangier and lighter.

### SERVES 2

about 150ml (5fl oz) mango pulp or purée (if using some from a large can, you can freeze any left over)
about 100ml (3½fl oz) chilled low-fat natural yogurt or, better still, milk kefir (see page 112 for homemade)
Cardamom Syrup (see page 14), to sweeten (optional)
a wedge of fresh mango, to serve (optional)

Spoon the mango pulp or purée into a bowl and add the yogurt or milk kefir. Taste, adding more mango or yogurt/kefir according to your preference (I personally like about half and half if I'm using kefir) and a little cardamom syrup to sweeten if you feel it needs it (I generally don't). Mix in enough water to make a drinking consistency.

Divide the lassi between two glasses and serve, with a wedge of fresh mango if you have some.

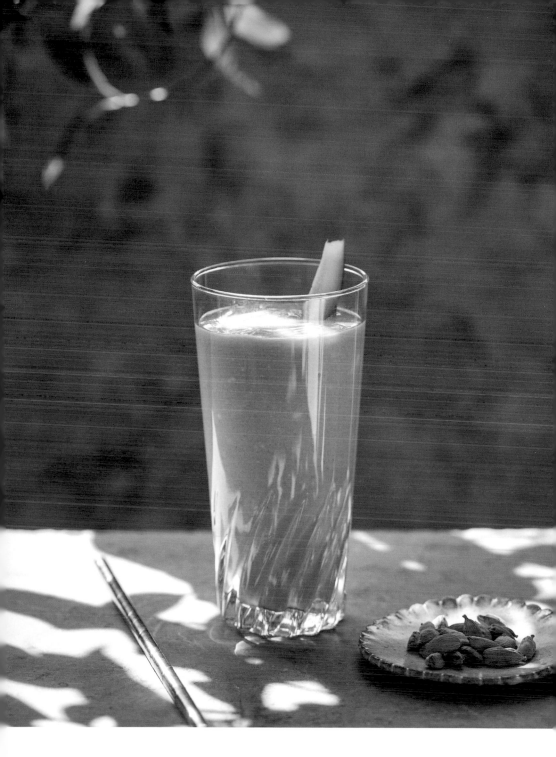

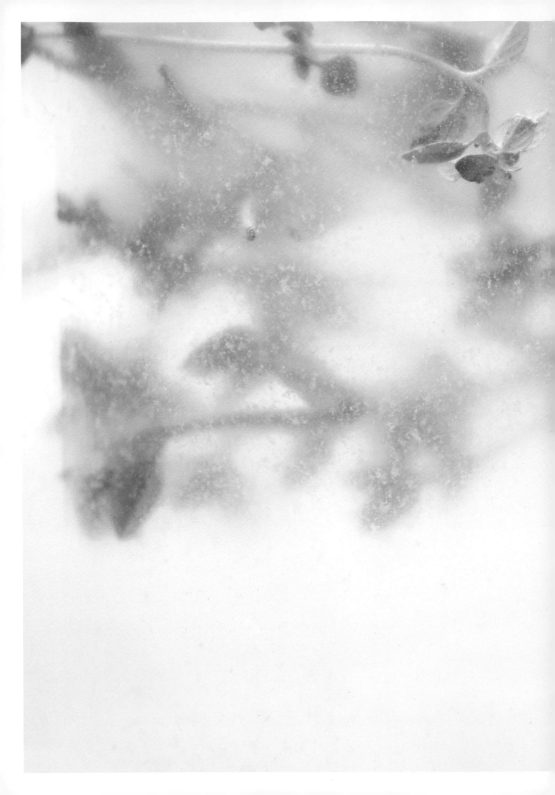

# JUICES AND
# SMOOTHIES

Juices and smoothies are nothing new, I know. I had a massive juicing phase in the '90s when I juiced every day and bounced around like Tigger as a result. We were all into it. It had nothing to do with whether you drank alcohol or not, frankly. In fact, it probably made it more likely that you would drink on account of feeling so darn healthy all the time. The only downside was the hassle of cleaning the juicer afterwards. Fibres would resolutely stick and sometimes remain embedded in the mesh filter. It really was a pain.

Now juicing has been given a new lease of life by popular appliances such as the Nutribullet and other "personal blenders" which are infinitely easier to use as they zhush up everything at the same time, thus combining the virtues of juicing with the ease of making smoothies. We've also learned that it's A Bad Thing to only juice fruit, which tends to give too much of a sugar rush (hence, presumably, all the bouncing), but that you should include some veg, preferably green veg, with it. I'm a bit ambivalent about that, partly because of the taste – greens like rocket and watercress can be bitter – but also the colour. It's easy to end up with an unappetising khaki sludge, though my pal Monica's pear and avocado smoothie is delicious.

Her advice, being a bit of an expert juicer and smoothie maker (you can find some of her recipes on her website smarterfitter.com) is to incorporate nutritious ingredients, such as nuts, seeds and grains, as an extra source of protein (which can obviously take the place of dairy if you're vegan) and dried fruit instead of added sweetener, though I must confess I like a bit of agave syrup or honey myself – and I don't have a particularly sweet tooth.

It's also worth learning which fruits and vegetables go naturally well together, both from the point of view of flavour and texture, so you can run up a juice or smoothie without having to think too much about it. Carrot and apple, for example, are both hard or hard-ish ingredients, but complement each other perfectly, along with celery if you fancy it. (Celery haters, you can't really taste it.) Strawberries and watermelon are perfectly matched, too, as are pineapple, mango and lime.

Don't be afraid either to include a ready-made juice for speed and sometimes a better flavour. I laboured long and hard with the Apple and Saffron Sharbat (see page 159), having been inspired by a similar drink in a restaurant, then found a shop-bought juice was the answer, as it was with the Beetroot and Pomegranate "Pinot" (see page 150).

Obviously juices and smoothies are not a substitute for alcohol – there are better alternatives in the other sections – but they're an extra and nutritious string to your bow. And hopefully satisfying and delicious enough to subdue that craving for a drink or even an impulsive high-calorie snack.

# Pineapple, Mango and Lime Juice

One of my all-time favourite juices. This is one of those perfect, unimprovable combinations of ingredients – but both the pineapple and mango need to be ripe.

**SERVES 4**

1 small–medium ripe
  pineapple
1 large ripe mango
1–2 limes

Peel the pineapple and remove the hard core, then cut up into pieces that will fit the feeder tube of your juicer. Peel and stone the mango, then cut up. Peel and cut up the limes.

Juice the pineapple and mango alternately, then finish with the lime. Alternatively, place the ingredients in a Nutribullet or similar personal blender with 75ml (5 tablespoons) water and blitz.

Divide the juice between four glasses and serve, garnished with a wedge of pineapple if you want to pretty it up.

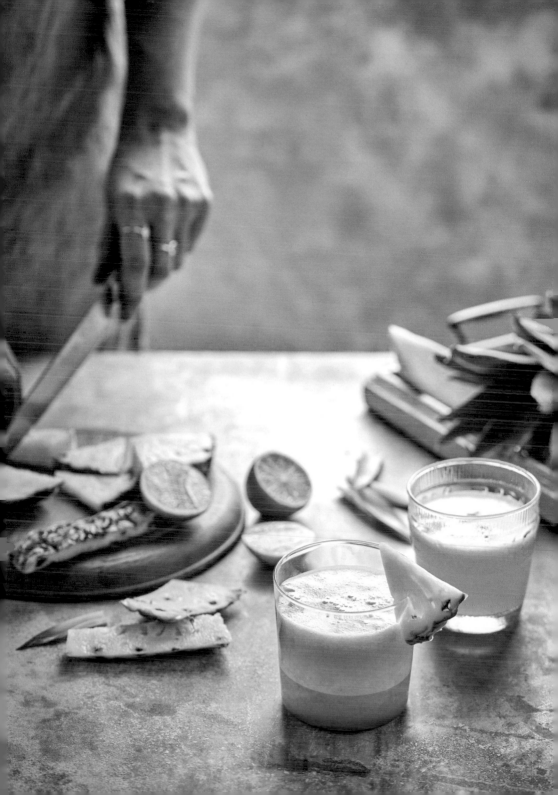

# Beetroot and Pomegranate "Pinot"

The biggest challenge if you're a wine lover is to find a drink that will be a decent substitute for red wine – something that has some body and structure to it but is not too sweet. This is the nearest I've got to it. Beetroot is not everyone's cup of tea, admittedly, but it has the richness and colour – a magnificent magenta if you make it with freshly juiced beets – to make you feel like you're enjoying a gutsy red. (See also page 190 for other drinks that do duty for red wine.) *Pictured on pages 152–153.*

MAKES 500ML (18FL OZ);
SERVES 4–6

250ml (9fl oz) freshly made
 beetroot juice (see below)
250ml (9fl oz) chilled good-
 quality pomegranate juice
 (I use POM Wonderful)
2 teaspoons balsamic
 vinegar, or to taste

Pour the beetroot and pomegranate juices into a jug and mix together, then add the vinegar to taste. The mixture tends to be a bit frothy to begin with, so if you want it to look more wine-like, pour it into a glass bottle or other container, stopper and let it rest in the refrigerator for a few hours before serving.

*\* Juicing beetroot: You'll need a bunch of fresh beetroot, about 450–500g (1lb–1lb 2oz) once you've removed the leaves. Peel the beets, using disposable plastic gloves if you want to avoid staining your hands crimson, and cut into pieces small enough to feed into the tube of your juicer. Juice following the manufacturer's instructions.*

# Carrot and Apple Juice

Carrot and apple is the juice everyone starts with and you can hardly better it. The exact balance will depend on what type of apples you use, but opt for organic produce where you can. *Pictured on pages 152–153*.

**SERVES 2**

2 medium or 3 small
   flavoursome apples
   (Cox's are ideal)
4 carrots
½ lemon (optional)

Cut the apples into quarters or pieces that will fit the feeder tube of your juicer. Trim and scrub the carrots, then cut up as necessary. Peel the lemon (if using), removing as much of the white pith as possible, and cut up.

Push the lemon through the feeder tube alternately with the apples and carrots. Alternatively, blitz together with 75ml (5 tablespoons) water in a Nutribullet or similar personal blender.

Divide the juice between two glasses and serve.

*VARIATION: SPICED CARROT, APPLE AND CELERY JUICE*
*Juice a celery stick along with the other ingredients and replace the lemon with a small cube of peeled fresh root ginger.*

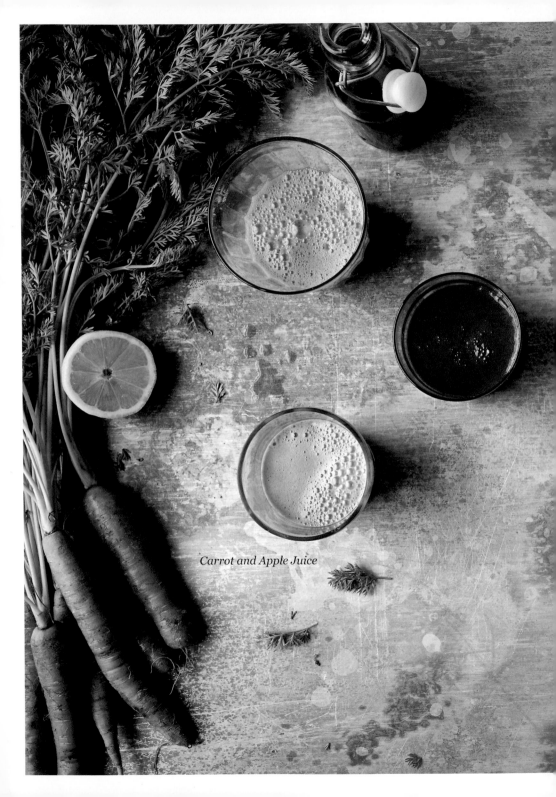

*Carrot and Apple Juice*

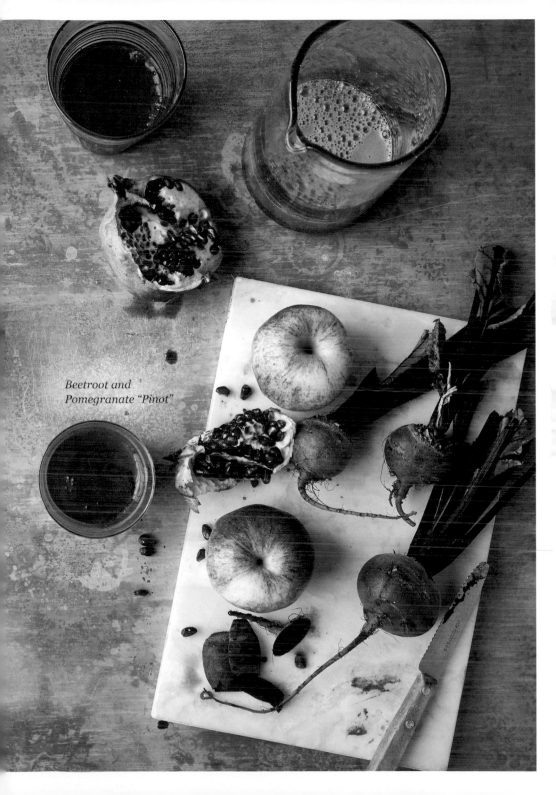

*Beetroot and Pomegranate "Pinot"*

# Strawberry Sunrise

This is one of the first smoothies I ever made and one I still love. The ingredients go so perfectly together. Best made in summer when locally-grown strawberries are in season, obviously.

**SERVES 2**

225g (8oz) ripe strawberries, plus extra to garnish
1 ripe banana
freshly squeezed juice of 1 orange
100ml (3½fl oz) natural yogurt or milk kefir
clear honey or agave syrup, to taste

Hull and halve the strawberries. Peel and slice the banana. Add the fruit to a blender with the orange juice and blend until smooth. Add the yogurt and honey or agave syrup to taste and blend again.

Divide the smoothie between two glasses and serve, topped with a slice of strawberry.

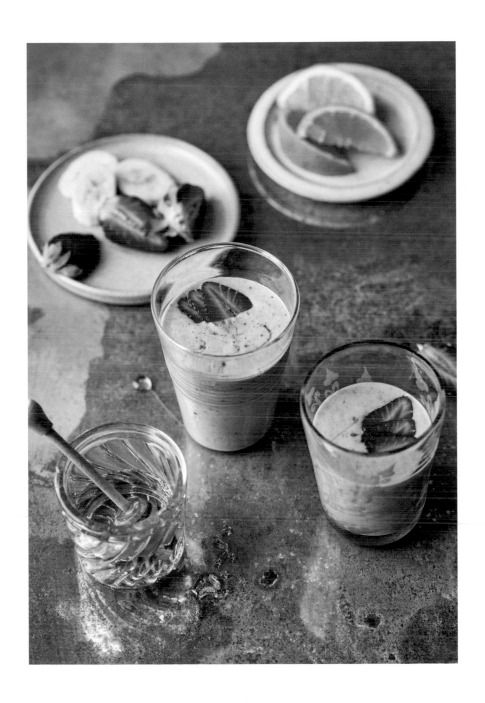

# Blueberry, Pear and Cinnamon Smoothie

Blueberries have such a wonderful colour that I can't really bear to diminish it with other ingredients, so this is a really simple smoothie. It's based on a bag of frozen blueberries, which work just as well as, if not better than, fresh ones.

**SERVES 1–2**

1 ripe medium-sized pear,
   quartered, cored and
   peeled
1 tablespoon lemon juice
100g (3½oz) frozen or fresh
   blueberries
100ml (3½fl oz) Greek
   yogurt or soy yogurt
a pinch of ground cinnamon
honey or agave syrup, to
   sweeten (optional)

Put the pear in a blender with the lemon juice, blueberries, yogurt and cinnamon. Add enough water to get the mixture moving (about 75ml/5 tablespoons). Whizz until smooth. If the blueberries are a bit tart, you can add a little honey or agave syrup, to taste.

Pour into 1–2 glass(es) to serve.

# Pear and Avocado Smoothie

Like most people I suspect, I think of smoothies as concoctions of delicious fruit, but I was put right by my friend Monica Shaw of smarterfitter.com, who insisted that for balance they should contain an element of veg. In this recipe she matches fresh pear with avocado, which go really well together. The avocado combined with the flaxseeds make this smoothie super thick and creamy. You can substitute other seeds or nuts for the flaxseeds, or omit completely if you don't have any to hand.

Taste aside, this smoothie contains a good balance of nutrients to make it wholesome, with loads of fibre provided by the pear, flaxseeds and leafy greens, healthy fats and delicious creaminess from the avocado, plus lemon for aiding digestion.

SERVES 1

1 large ripe pear, peeled
  and cored
½ ripe avocado, peeled and
  stoned
¼ small lemon, peeled and
  white pith removed
handful of kale or spinach
2 pitted dates (optional)
1 heaped teaspoon
  flaxseeds
a few ice cubes
pinch of salt

Add all the ingredients to a powerful blender or food processor, including the dates if you prefer a slightly sweeter smoothie, along with a little bit of water. Start blending and add more water to taste, depending how thick you like your smoothie.

Pour into a tall glass and serve.

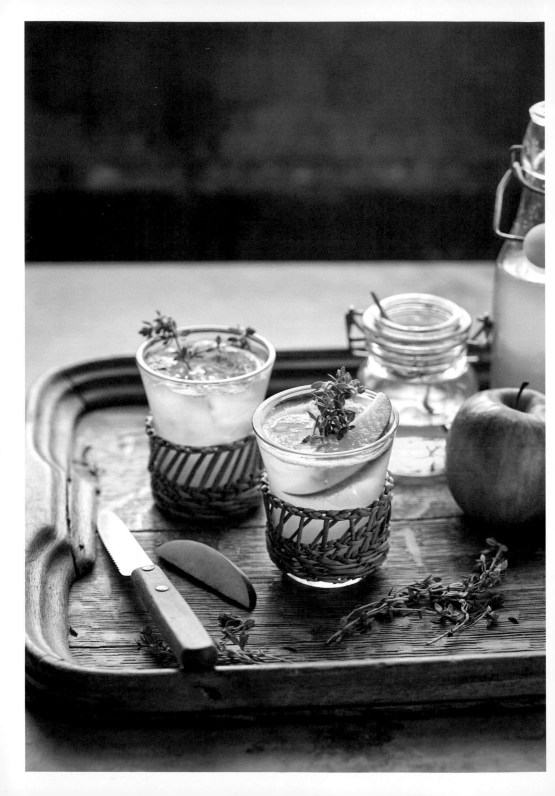

# Apple and Saffron Sharbat

I discovered this utterly delicious drink in a Persian restaurant called Berenjak in London's Soho and badgered them about it until they revealed that the base cordial was made by one of my favourite soft drink producers, Square Root London (see page 186). They, of course, make it from scratch using fresh ingredients, and you may want to do likewise, but it does involve a lot of juicing, particularly if you make it in quantity, and the problem with apples is that they easily discolour. So I found you could cheat really effectively using a shop-bought cloudy apple juice. If you have an apple glut, though, it makes sense to use fresh fruit. The saffron infusion yields slightly more than you need, but you can strain and refrigerate it and experiment with adding it to other drinks.

**SERVES 3–4**

small pinch of saffron
   threads (about 10)
3 tablespoons warm water
450ml (16fl oz) unsweetened
   cloudy apple juice or juice
   from freshly juiced apples
   – Robyn of Square Root
   (see recipe introduction)
   says they use a mixture of
   cooking and eating apples
about 1 tablespoon freshly
   squeezed lemon juice
about 1 tablespoon Sugar
   Syrup (see page 14)
generous splash of sparkling
   water
ice cubes
sprigs of thyme, to garnish

Put the saffron in a small bowl, cover with the measured warm water and leave to infuse for 15 minutes or so. Strain and leave to cool.

Pour the apple juice into a jug and add about one tablespoon each of the saffron infusion, lemon juice and sugar syrup, adjusting the mixture to taste, although be cautious with the saffron, as it's easy to overdo it. Add a good splash of sparkling water.

Fill three or four glasses with ice, pour over the sharbat, garnish with sprigs of thyme and serve.

# Citron Pressé

This French café classic is one of the easiest ways to enjoy a juice (though see Orange Kefir Water, page 115, which is equally delicious).

**SERVES 1**

1 lemon
1–2 teaspoons granulated
  sugar, to taste
chilled water

Cut the lemon in half, squeeze the juice and pour it into a glass. (You can strain it if you prefer, but I seldom bother.)

Sweeten to taste with the sugar, top up with chilled water and serve.

# Green Gazpacho

This recipe is the result of a fridge forage – just imagine all your salad ingredients in a glass (but gazpacho sounds much more sexy, don't you think?). You can vary it depending on the ingredients you have available, but don't overdo the tomatoes or it might turn an unattractive sludge colour. It's easiest to make this in a personal blender like a Nutribullet, but a conventional blender will do.

## SERVES 1

Little Gem lettuce leaves, preferably the paler crunchy ones, torn
¼ to ⅓ cucumber, chopped
1 spring onion, trimmed and chopped, or a handful of chives
1 medium tomato, quartered
a handful of seedless green grapes
a few sprigs of parsley or dill (optional)
1 tablespoon lemon juice
sea salt, to taste

Put the torn lettuce leaves in the blender goblet with the cucumber, spring onion or chives, tomato, grapes, herbs (if using) and lemon juice. Add enough water to reach halfway up the ingredients (or up to the "Max" mark if you're using a Nutribullet) and season with sea salt.

Whizz until smooth. Pour into a tall glass and serve.

Tip: You could also add a shake of Tabasco mild green pepper sauce to make it a touch spicier, if you like.

*VARIATION: GREEN GAZPACHO SHOTS*
*The recipe above makes a thick, pulpy juice.*
*To make green gazpacho shots, strain the juice and pour it into shot glasses for a fresh, green hit.*

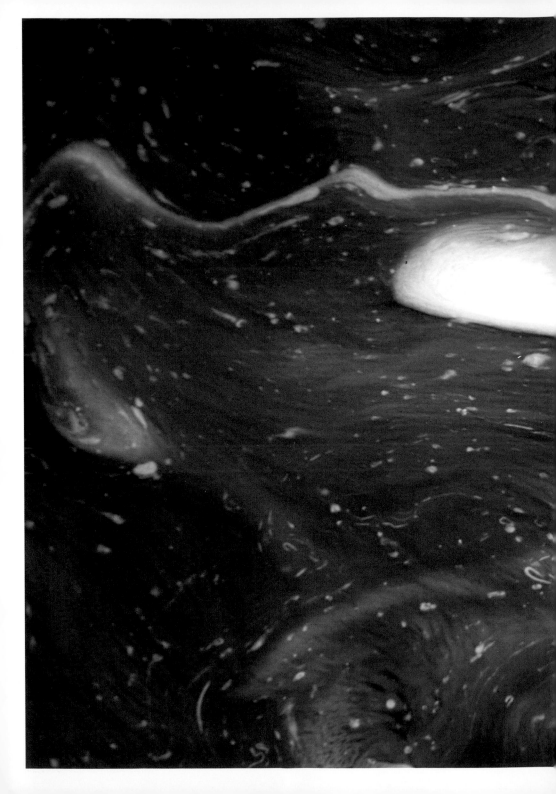

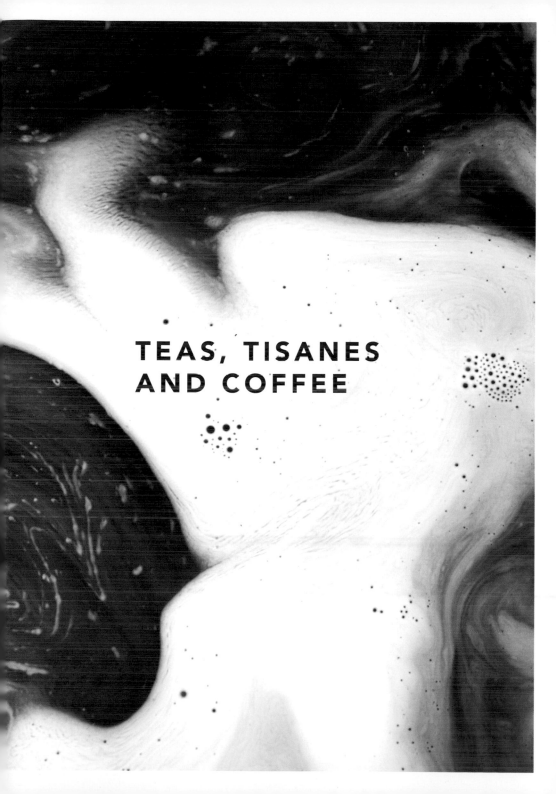

# TEAS, TISANES AND COFFEE

Coffee and tea are by far the most interesting alternatives to alcohol unless you have the misfortune to be sensitive to caffeine. Even then you can get really good decaffeinated coffee these days and there's a wide range of herbal teas and infusions to enjoy.

Both coffee and tea involve the kind of geekery in terms of different leaves, beans and origins that makes wine so fascinating, not to mention endless bits of interesting kit. And they go really well with food once you get used to the idea of doing without alcohol. Much better than most soft drinks, if truth be told.

Let's start with tea. There's a fair chance that you're not getting the best out of the tea you're drinking because you're making it too quickly (blame tea bags) and brewing it at the wrong temperature. I always wondered why I had such an aversion to green tea until I discovered that pouring boiling water over it enhances its bitterness and makes it taste like grass clippings. (You should brew it at 80°C/176°F). White tea and oolong (my favourite) need to be made with water that's off the boil, too. So either leave your water to cool or, better still, get a kettle with different temperature settings.

I don't need to tell you that tea is far better made from loose leaves than the powdery dust found in the average tea bag. But you'll get a much more enjoyable experience if you pour all the liquid off the leaves rather than leaving it to stew, then re-infuse them when you want another cup. With good-quality teas you can do that several times, which will make you feel virtuously frugal. There are various kinds of infusers on the market which are easier to use than a pot if you're just making tea for one.

Your coffee habit may also need rethinking, even if you've acquired yourself a Nespresso or similar smart coffee machine. I was so stuck in my espresso habit that it came as a massive surprise to find that filter coffee, which I'd always derided, could reveal the character of a particular bean at least as well as, if not better than, an espresso shot, particularly if made with freshly ground beans. I actually went on a course with a local coffee company, Extract Coffee in Bristol, UK, to improve my coffee making technique and acquired, as a result, an electric coffee grinder, although you don't even need that if you have a good coffee shop nearby which will grind your beans for you, and a simple, inexpensive V60 drip filter. As a result, I've discovered the kind of coffee I most enjoy – fragrant brews from Ethiopia and Rwanda. You also learn how quickly coffee goes off and that you need to buy coffee little and often to enjoy it at its best.

Cold brew is also transformative. I assumed it would be harsh and bitter, but the reverse is true. It's rich and velvety, as you'll discover if you follow the recipe on page 179. Truly, tea and coffee can be just as absorbing as beer, whisky and wine.

# Fresh Herbal Teas or Tisanes

Fresh herb teas or tisanes are so very much nicer than the dried versions you buy in tea bags (I especially hate dried mint). Here are my favourite five to try. Bear in mind that they're better made with water that has not quite come up to the boil – about 80°C (176°F) – so as not to scorch the delicate leaves.

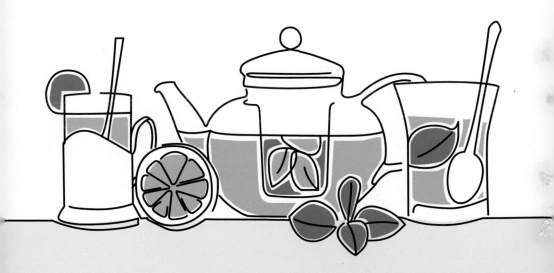

### FRESH MINT TEA

Basically mint leaves with hot water poured over them. Add a little sugar, if you like. When you're ordering this in restaurants, make sure to specify fresh mint tea, or they'll often serve you a peppermint tea bag (while still charging an outrageous amount for it).

### MOROCCAN MINT TEA

The Moroccan version is sweeter and a bit more sophisticated. Place a sprig of mint in a cup with a green tea bag and 1 teaspoon sugar. Pour over water that has not quite come up to the boil (see left) and leave to infuse for a couple of minutes. Remove the tea bag and stir to dissolve the sugar.

### VERVEINE

Reputed to aid digestion and promote relaxation, lemon verbena (or Verveine, as it's known in France, where it's hugely popular), is my favourite late-night drink. It's the one exception to my general rule that fresh leaves are infinitely better than dried, as dried lemon verbena will work fine, although it's better to use whole leaves rather than a tea bag. However, if you can find fresh lemon verbena leaves in the summer – or harvest fresh from your garden or patio container – they are delicious, with a heavenly lemon fragrance.

### ROSEMARY TEA

I have a friend who gives me this every time I go round to dinner, while her husband, who has no problem with sleeping, knocks back his espresso. It's simply a sprig of rosemary, preferably freshly picked, a quarter slice of lemon and ½ teaspoon of honey or agave syrup with hot water poured over it (in this case, you can use boiling water, as rosemary can take it).

### SAGE TEA

Slightly more bitter than rosemary, but with similar health benefits and bracingly refreshing. Infuse 8 large sage leaves in 225ml (8fl oz) hot water for 10 minutes. Sweeten with honey or agave syrup to taste.

# Bubble Tea

I wasn't really conscious of bubble tea when I started writing this book. But by the time I finished it, it seemed to be everywhere, perhaps not coincidentally given that my hometown of Bristol in the UK has a large Chinese student community. However, it seems to be incredibly popular among pre-teen and teenage girls, too.

If it isn't on your radar, bubble tea is very popular in China and all over Southeast Asia. It's basically tea to which either milk or fruit juice, tapioca pearls and occasionally popping fruit jellies are added, creating a colourful and generally sweet drink that you sip through a giant straw, chewing the bubbles as they emerge.

In the best bubble tea bars, the tea is freshly brewed and mixed with fresh fruit juice or milk, traditionally cows' milk, but dairy-free alternatives are widely available. Although there are a huge number of variations, you can also ask for your tea to be tailored to your own personal taste – made sweeter or less sweet, or with or without toppings, for example.

Think of the fruit-based bubble teas as a souped-up juice and the milk ones more like a latte-type drink or shake. In fact, the term bubble tea originally referred to the froth you create by shaking it, not the tapioca pearls.

You can make bubble tea at home – you simply need to buy some tapioca pearls or *boba*, which you can find in Chinese and other Asian supermarkets, but you have to cook them and it's hard to achieve exactly the right consistency. And as with flat whites, part of the fun is the theatre of watching the bubble tea baristas (if there is such a thing) make them to order.

What's interesting about the bubble tea phenomenon is that it creates a colourful caffeine-free – or largely caffeine-free – alternative to coffee shops and alcohol-free alternative cocktail bars, cementing the appeal of the sober lifestyle among younger consumers.

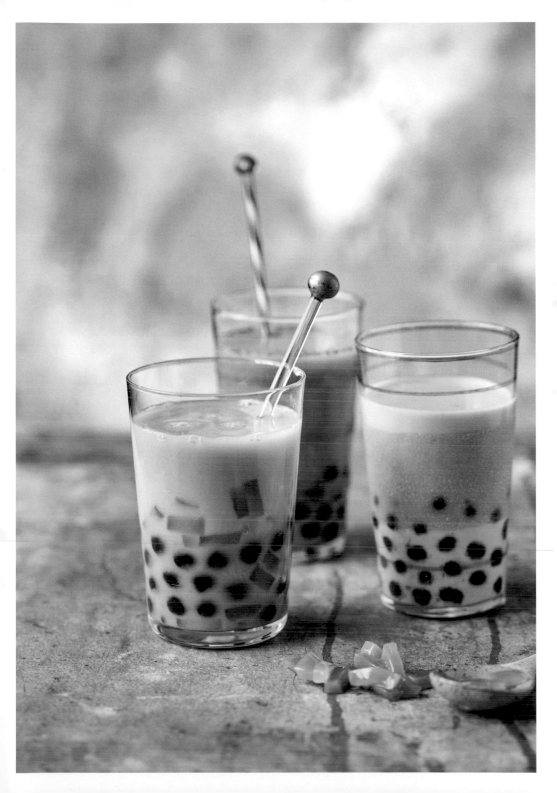

# Hibiscus Agua Fresca

You can buy dried hibiscus flowers, also known as Jamaica flowers, in Mexican and Caribbean grocery stores, as well as from online suppliers. *Pictured on page 172.*

SERVES 1

handful of ice cubes
50ml (2fl oz) Hibiscus Syrup (see below)
sparkling water, to top up
wedge of lime
slice of lime or 2 poached hibiscus flowers (reserved from making the Hibiscus Syrup), to garnish

FOR THE HIBISCUS SYRUP (MAKES 750ML/1⅓ PINTS)
100g (3½oz) granulated or caster sugar
850ml (1½ pints) water
20g (¾oz) dried hibiscus flowers
juice of 1 lime

To make the hibiscus syrup, put the sugar in a saucepan and add the measured water. Heat over a low heat, stirring occasionally, until the sugar has dissolved. Bring to the boil and add the hibiscus flowers, then simmer for about 30 minutes. Take off the heat and stir in the lime juice, then cover and leave to infuse for 30 minutes.

Strain the contents of the pan through a fine sieve into a wide-necked jug or bowl, then pour the liquid through a funnel into a sterilized 75cl bottle. Leave to cool, seal and store in the refrigerator for up to 2 weeks.

Drop a handful of ice cubes into a tumbler. Pour in the hibiscus syrup and top up with sparkling water. Squeeze the wedge of lime into the drink, drop it into the glass and stir. Garnish with a couple of the poached hibiscus flowers and serve.

# Golden Turmeric Tea

For this I like to use the fresh root rather than ground turmeric. The tea is not as effective as the Turmeric Latte (see page 128) as a source of curcumin, the active ingredient in turmeric that contains all the health-giving properties, as it doesn't contain either black pepper or fat, but it makes a fresher-tasting drink as a result. I strongly advise using disposable plastic gloves to grate the turmeric unless you want to have yellow-stained fingers for the rest of the day. *Pictured on page 173.*

**SERVES 2**

1 fresh turmeric root, washed
2.5cm (1-inch) piece of fresh ginger, peeled
3 strips of finely pared unwaxed lemon rind
300ml (10fl oz) hot water
honey or agave syrup, to taste

Grate the turmeric and ginger into a small saucepan, add the lemon rind and pour over the measured hot water. Leave to infuse for 10 minutes.

Strain the infusion and reheat in a microwave oven if you have one, or use a small pan if you don't. Sweeten to taste with honey or agave syrup (I think honey works better in this recipe unless you have an objection to using it). You can then infuse the turmeric and ginger again, if you like, to make a further batch of tea.

Divide between two cups or heatproof glasses and serve.

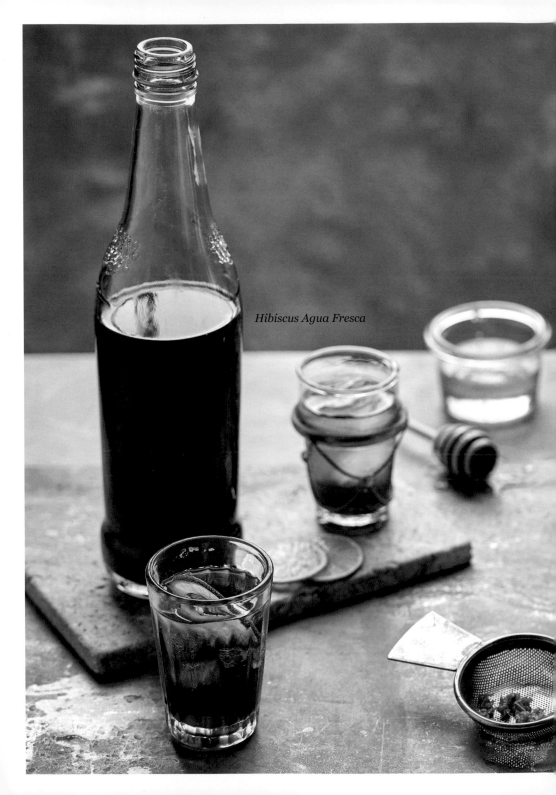

*Hibiscus Agua Fresca*

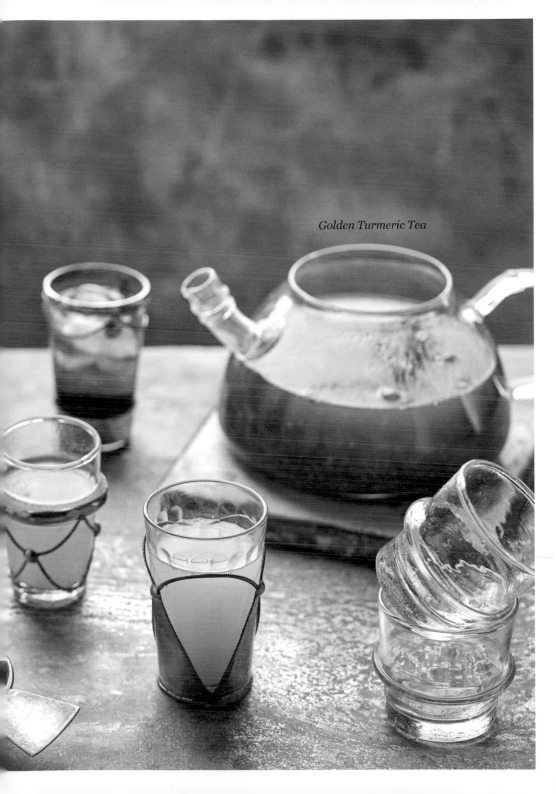

*Golden Turmeric Tea*

# Cold Brew Tea

You might think you wouldn't get much flavour out of tea that's been brewed in cold water – I didn't either and I was amazed. It's particularly well suited to delicate teas like green tea that can be scorched and made to taste bitter by boiling water. It's also mercifully sugar-free, although you will add a little when you top it up with tonic to serve (see T&T, page 176). Make up a jug and keep it in the refrigerator.

**MAKES ABOUT 400ML (14FL OZ)**

3 tea bags (I like Earl Grey green tea bags) or 2–3 teaspoons loose tea, depending on the tea (a stronger brew than usual, but you're going to be diluting it with ice to serve)
400ml (14fl oz) water

Put the tea bags or tea leaves in a jug or other container, pour over the measured water and stir. Cover and leave to brew at room temperature for 5–6 hours, or in the refrigerator overnight, before serving.

**Tip:** Fill a flask with cold brew tea and carry it with you when you're on the move. It's much cheaper – and nicer – than the commercial cold-infuse tea bags.

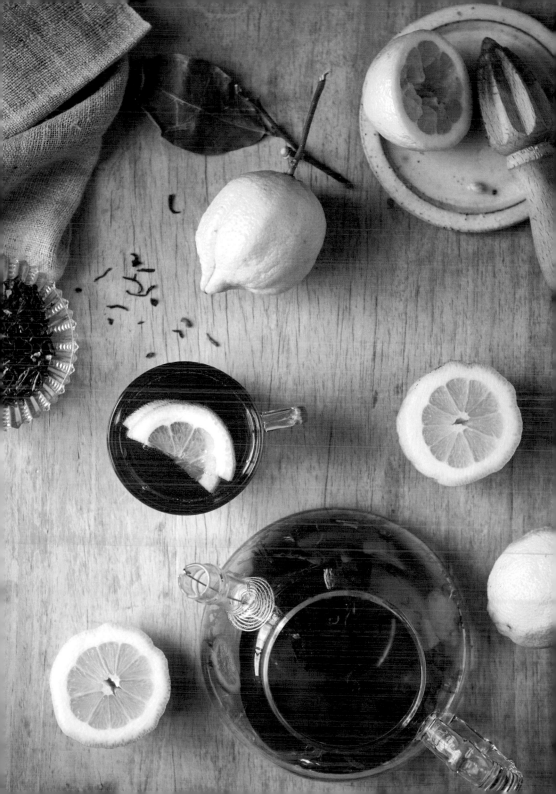

# T&T

Tea and tonic: a perfect drink for that gin and tonic moment if you don't have an alcohol-free spirit to hand, or don't want to go down the juniper syrup route.

**SERVES 1**

ice cubes
about 200ml (7fl oz) strained Cold Brew Tea (see page 174)
generous squeeze of lemon, about 5ml (1 teaspoon)
splash of Indian tonic water, to top up
slice of lemon, to garnish

Fill a tumbler with ice cubes. Pour over the cold brew tea, squeeze in the lemon juice and stir to mix. Top up with a splash of Indian tonic water.

Garnish with a slice of lemon and serve.

# Rooibos Tea Punch

Like the Quince, Honey and Lemon Cordial on page 34 and the Rhubarb Cordial on page 39, this is another dual purpose recipe that generates a fruit compote as well as a drink, in this case rather like the German *rumtopf* but without the rum, obviously. The colour will depend on the amount of prunes you have in the mix. Prunes tend to make it a rather murky brown, though the drink gets lighter as you dilute it. If you want it to be lighter still, stick to dried apples, pears and peaches or apricots.

**MAKES ABOUT 750ML (1⅓ PINTS) TEA PUNCH,** *PLUS 4 SERVINGS OF DRIED FRUIT COMPOTE*

3 rooibos tea bags
750ml (1⅓ pints) water just off the boil
250g (9oz) mixed dried fruit
40g (1½oz) light muscovado sugar
cinnamon stick
finely pared strip of unwaxed orange rind (optional)
water, to serve

Put the tea bags in a teapot or heatproof jug, pour over the measured hot water and leave to brew for about 7–8 minutes.

Put the dried fruit in a saucepan with the sugar, cinnamon and orange rind, if using. Pour over the rooibos tea, discarding the tea bags, stir and bring to the boil, then simmer for about 20 minutes until the fruit is soft. Take off the heat and leave for a further 30 minutes to infuse.

Strain the contents of the pan through a fine sieve into a wide-necked jug or bowl. Transfer what is now in essence a dried fruit compote with a little of the juice to moisten. Then pour the remaining juice through a funnel into a sterilized 75cl bottle. Leave to cool, seal and store in the refrigerator up to 2 weeks.

To serve, dilute the punch to taste with water.

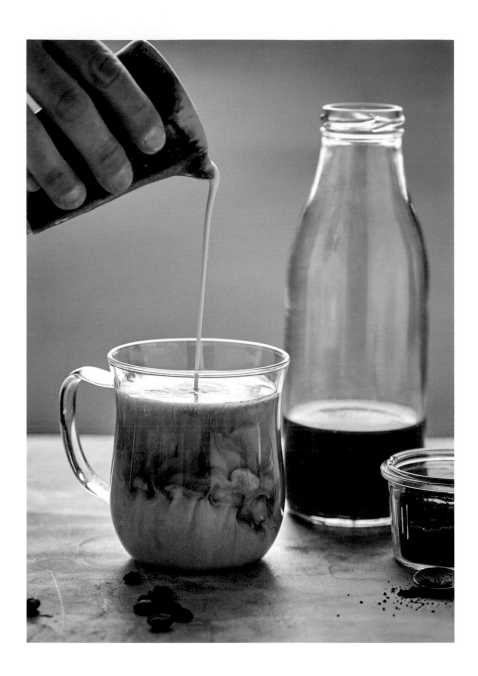

# Iced Cold Brew Coffee

Cold brew coffee is a revelation if you haven't tried it before, especially if you generally find coffee too bitter and extracted. The long infusion of the grounds creates a rich, dark, velvety drink that reveals the character of the individual beans much more effectively than most brewing methods.

**SERVES 2**

30g (1oz) roasted coffee beans, ideally freshly roasted
250ml (9fl oz) cold filtered water or still mineral water
ice cubes
1–2 teaspoons Sugar Syrup (see page 14) or hazelnut or other flavoured coffee syrup, to taste (optional)
dairy single cream or non-dairy alternative, to taste

Grind the coffee beans on the coarsest setting on your coffee grinder. Put them in a cafetière, pour over the measured filtered or mineral water and stir to mix. Cover without plunging and leave to infuse for at least 12 and up to 20 hours.

Steadily depress the plunger and pour the coffee through a muslin-lined fine sieve into a wide-necked jug (if serving soon) or a sterilized bottle. Cover or seal and store in the refrigerator for up to 2 weeks.

When you're ready to serve, fill two small glasses with ice, pour over the coffee and add the sugar syrup or flavoured syrup to taste, then trickle in some single cream or a non-dairy alternative.

To serve cold brew as a hot drink, simply heat it in a microwave or saucepan until just below simmering point. It will still retain that rounded velvety taste.

---

*VARIATION: VIETNAMESE-STYLE COFFEE*
*You can also serve your cold brew coffee, or any other black coffee, Vietnamese-style by heating up about 150ml (5fl oz) and pouring it slowly into a glass, into which you've added 2 tablespoons condensed milk. If you pour steadily, the coffee should float rather picturesquely on top of the milk until you stir it in, creating a sweet, slightly caramelly brew.*

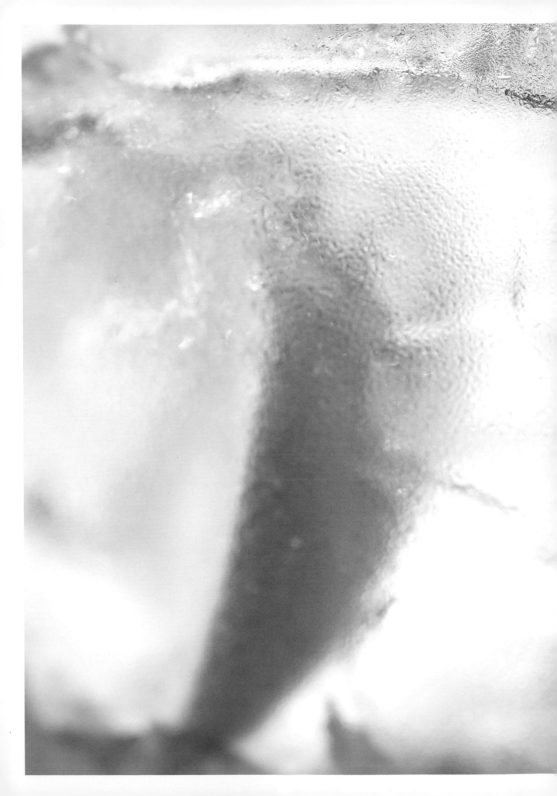

# WHAT TO
# DRINK WHEN

# 50 OF THE BEST ALCOHOL-FREE BRANDS AND DRINKS

For those of you who don't want to make your own drinks, or are looking for an alternative to an alcoholic drink you enjoy, the good news is that there's an absolute deluge of NOLO (no- and low-alcohol) products arriving on the market currently – some 80 spirit substitutes alone at the time of writing. So this list will almost certainly not take account of all of them, but these are the ones that have impressed me most while I've been researching this book.

### ALCOHOL-FREE BEERS

*Beer is the star of the show so far as alcohol-free alternatives to conventional booze are concerned, which is no surprise given that the main flavouring ingredients – malt and hops – are still present. I'd ignore the big brands' offerings and look at what the craft brewers have to offer.*

### BrewDog Nanny State (0.5% ABV)
You'd have expected trendsetters Brewdog to jump on the NOLO bandwagon and they were first out of the traps with this cannily named pale ale substitute. It's usefully widely available, too.

### Mikkeller Drink'in the Sun (0.3% ABV)
The name says it all – fragrant, hoppy and packed with passion fruit and citrus. The perfect summer beer from this innovative Danish craft brewer.

### Big Drop Brewing Co.
Set up specifically to brew alcohol-free beers. I like their pale ale and stout best. Cool labels, too.

### Thornbridge Big Easy (0.5% ABV)
Superbly fresh, hoppy and happy-making beer from this excellent Derbyshire brewery in the East Midlands of England.

### Nirvana Kosmic Stout (0% ABV)
Dark, full-flavoured, chocolatey and gluten-free. My favourite of their range.

### Lucky Saint (0.5% ABV)
The best lager I've come across so far, though hoppier and spicier than more commercial versions. Unfiltered.

## ALCOHOL-FREE CIDERS

*Slightly harder to nail than beer, not least in balancing the sweetness, but they're getting better.*

### Sheppy's Low Alcohol Classic Cider (0.5% ABV)

Crisp and fruity – a decent cider alternative from a traditional Somerset cider maker.

### Braxzz Oaked Cider

Completely alcohol-free full-flavoured cider developed by a Dutch brewery and made in Germany.

## ALCOHOL-FREE WINES

*Unless you're permanently avoiding alcohol, I can't really recommend alcohol-free wines, particularly reds – they simply don't cut the mustard if you're a wine lover. But if you yearn for a glass of fizz or an aromatic white, you may find them acceptable.*

### Natureo Muscat (0% ABV)

Far-sighted Spanish producer Torres started making alcohol-free wines back in 2008 and this fragrant Muscat would easily do duty for a Riesling or Gewürztraminer. Perfect with stir-fries and other spicy food.

### Botonique (0% ABV)

Intended as a substitute for prosecco, but with a herbal flavour more akin to a vermouth. It may be a touch bitter for some.

### The Bees Knees Alcohol-Free Sparkling Rosé (0% ABV)

A little sweet for my palate, but one of the better AF sparkling wines out there.

### Rawson's Retreat

The main NOLO player from Down Under. I like their sparkling Chardonnay Pinot Noir Muscat (0.5% ABV) best. It's a little sweeter and fruitier than a standard sparkling wine – more like a fruit cocktail, but actually quite pleasant.

### Outfox White Sauvignon (0.5% ABV)

In its stylish opaque white bottle, this Sauvignon wannabe should appeal if you're a New Zealand Sauvignon Blanc fan.

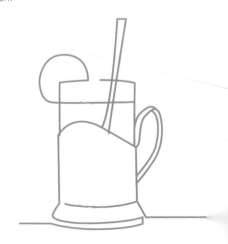

## ALCOHOL-FREE SPIRITS

### Seedlip

Seedlip was the drink that kicked the whole alcohol-free spirits craze off. Packaged in stylish heavy glass bottles, they not only tasted like a gin but looked like one, too – with a price to match. There are three products in the range at the time of writing: Spice 94, which is the closest to gin; Garden 108, which is more summery and herbal; and Grove 42, which is citrussy and designed to be served with orange. All need to be diluted with tonic or soda water and I personally find they are generally better in a cocktail, though I was grateful to have them as a G&T substitute on Virgin Atlantic, who have taken them on as an alcohol-free option on their flights.

### Caleño

Invented by Columbian-born and Bristol-based Ellie Webb, this has more of a tropical taste, derived from Inca berries. Really rather delicious.

### Ceder's Alt-gin

Ceder's founders coined the phrase "alt-gin" to describe their non-alcoholic "spirits", which are made in Sweden with South African botanicals including bucho and rooibos. "Classic" is flavoured with juniper, coriander and rose geranium, while "Crisp" has extracts of cucumber and chamomile.

### Strykk

Strykk has a wider range including an alternative to rum (Not Rum), Not Gin and a cucumbery Not Vodka, which is my own favourite. With their bright, jazzy labels, they consciously target younger 18–35-year-old consumers who choose not to drink. Cheaper than some of the other "spirits", too.

## APERITIFS

### Aecorn

Really convincing alternatives to vermouth from the Seedlip stable, though launched as a separate brand. Includes Aromatic, which is flavoured with smoked cherry wood and cloves, Dry (more herbal – like a dry vermouth) and Bitter, which is infused with quassia and gentian. The best substitute for classic cocktails like a Negroni or Americano.

### Everleaf

Sophisticated citrussy aperitif created by biologist Paul Mathew, whose father worked at the Royal Botanic Gardens, Kew (UK) and wrote the definitive books on two of Everleaf's ingredients, Crocus and Iris. Designed to be diluted with soda water.

### Crodino

A really convincing alternative to the Aperol Spritz – made by the same company (which also makes Campari).

You can serve it simply over ice with a slice of orange (and a fat green olive if you have one), but I generally add a splash of soda water, too.

## Monte Rosso

Another good, bittersweet Italian-style aperitivo flavoured with rowan berries and wild cranberries and blended with bitters and soda water. Serve over ice with a slice of orange.

## Rocktails Citrus Spritz

Flavoured with lemon, grapefruit and lavender – a sophisticated, dry, herby, citrussy aperitif.

## TONICS AND OTHER MIXERS

### Fever-Tree

Move over Schweppes - Fever-Tree is now the main game in town when it comes to tonic, although I do find their standard Indian tonic water a touch sweet. (In general, the Refreshingly Light range is . . . er . . . lighter). Where they excel though, especially if you're looking to drink them on their own, is with their flavoured tonics. I'm a big fan of the Aromatic and Mediterranean tonics in their standard range, cucumber rocks my boat in the summer and clementine tonic in the winter. And elderflower, of course, if you're an elderflower fan (it is slightly less sweet than elderflower cordial).

## Merchant's Heart Pink Peppercorn

I sometimes find flavoured tonics, or "spirit enhancers" as we must now call them, too complex for gin, but again they're great on their own. The Merchant's Heart Pink Peppercorn being a case in point.

## Luscombe Cool and Hot Ginger Beer

Luscombe has morphed from selling classically English drinks, such as apple juice and lemonade, to producing a wide range of mixers. I particularly like their ginger beer which comes in cool and hot versions. (The cool version is delicious with Rhubarb Cordial, page 39.)

## London Essence

Another company that spans mixers and soft drinks. I particularly like their Rhubarb and Cardamom Soda which does duty for a Provençal rosé (at least people will think that's what it is).

## Long Tail

Unusually, the Long Tail range is designed to go with dark rather than white spirits, which gives them a slightly different flavour profile from ones designed to go with gin. For drinking on their own, I like the Island Spice, a refreshing blend of chinotto (orange-type citrus fruit), gentian and spices, and the Ginger Lime.

## CORDIALS AND COCKTAIL MIXES

### Square Root London

My favourite cordial company both because they only use fresh ingredients and are always innovating. They make a delicious Non-alcoholic Gin & Tonic, which is flavoured, among other botanicals, with Persian dried lime, and collaborate with local London brewers to make very low alcohol (0.5%) shandies. They were also the inspiration for my Apple and Saffron Sharbat on page 159, which is loosely based on one they make for the Persian restaurant Berenjak in London's Soho.

### Monin

It's almost a question of is there a flavour that the French drinks producer Monin doesn't make, rather than listing what it does, which ranges from a lemon tart to a lavender syrup, which I've used in the Lavender Milk on page 138 as well as useful alcohol-free versions of cocktail ingredients like Triple Sec. You won't find them everywhere, but you can buy them online – from Amazon even, or, more cheaply from The Whisky Exchange.

### Teisseire Passion Fruit Sirop

You have to hand it to the French – they are good at cordials and their passion fruit sirop (which I've used in the Passionate Lady on page 63) is one I always try to have to hand. Try the Pink Grapefruit, too.

### Tipplesworth Espresso Martini Mixer

Designed to be mixed with booze, but just as good without it, though you may want to add an extra shot of espresso if you don't have a particularly sweet tooth.

### Bottle Green Aromatic Ginger and Lemongrass Cordial

A long established brand, better known for its elderflower cordial, but I prefer this punchy ginger and lemongrass version which is great with Chinese food. (Also good with an added squeeze of lime.)

## SHRUBS

*Personally, I prefer a homemade shrub (see pages 46–48) but there are a couple of brands on the market you should look out for.*

### Nonsuch Sour Cherry and Garden Mint

My favourite of the Nonsuch range, which is made by a member of the Aspall family which produces the cyder vinegar that goes into it. Sour cherry rocks!

### Wolfe's Pineapple, Chilli and Lime Leaf

An unusual shrub with a clearly defined pineapple flavour and a nice kick of chilli, but not too hot. Would be good with spicy or Caribbean food.

## JUICES

*A lot of cheap juices are made out of imported concentrate rather than freshly juiced fruit, so check the label carefully.*

### Biona

It's worth paying the extra for this premium organic blend, which has really natural flavours. I particularly like the elderberry which is a good substitute for red wine, and the grape juice, which is less sweet than many other brands, though I still like to add a dash of balsamic vinegar to it.

### Savsé Super Blue

As good as a homemade smoothie – not least because it includes a bit of veg (beetroot, spinach and kale) as well as fruit (it tastes of blueberry and blackcurrant, although it's based on apple juice). Cold-pressed, unpasteurized, no added sugar.

### Cawston Press Apple and Rhubarb

I like all the Cawston range with their very English flavours but particularly this for its extra touch of tartness. They conveniently come in cans, too.

### Woodstar Acai Berry Blend 1%

Not totally alcohol-free, but this tart French wine-like drink, which is based on Brazilian Acai berries (with added blueberries and cherries), is a good substitute for a light to medium bodied red wine.

### Big Tom Spiced Tomato Mix

Basically a ready-made Virgin Mary – and a good one – from fruit juice producer James White (whose apple juices are also good).

## FLAVOURED WATERS

*I'm not a big fan of flavoured waters – it's so easy to make your own at considerably less expense – but they are a thing. Here's a few names to look out for.*

### La Croix
Snappily packaged, sugar-free seltzer (sparkling water) that's become cult drinking among millennials in the US. Wide range of French-inspired flavours including cerise-limon (cherry lime) and melon pomelo (canteloupe melon and pink grapefruit).

### Dash Cucumber
An appealing range of sparkling spring waters infused with "wonky" fruit and veg that would otherwise go to waste. I particularly like the cucumber.

### Luscombe Sour Cherry Water
My cherry fetish on display again. A refreshing sparkling water made with organic fruit.

### No.1 Rosemary Water
Refreshingly herbal water for those who find fruit-flavoured waters too sweet. (A touch expensive, though, and you can make your own – see page 21.)

## KOMBUCHA
### Real Kombucha
One of the best kombucha ranges I've tasted made with quality teas – a great alternative to white wine or sake. My favourite is the Royal Flush, which is made with first flush Darjeeling, but Dry Dragon (green tea) and Smoke House (Yunnan) are also delicious.

### GT Organic and Raw Kombucha
One of the best known and most widely distributed brands in the US with many different flavours.

## KEFIR
### Biotiful Kefir Honey and Ginger Smoothie
Despite the cringe-making pun of a name, this is a really appealing drink with the edge taken off the tartness with a little honey. It's quite thick, so you might want to add a splash of water.

### Redwood Hill Farm Plain Kefir
Award-winning kefir from California made from organic goat's milk.

## DAIRY AND DAIRY-FREE
### Rebel Mylk
Pricier than most of the other non-dairy milks (it's a blend of organic coconut cream, brown rice and cashew), but with an exceptionally creamy taste and texture.

### Innocent Unsweetened Coconut
I wasn't going to include Innocent as they're sure to be on your radar already, but their new (at the time of writing) unsweetened coconut is delicious.

### Rude Health
A highly successful brand which started off making cereals (they're good, too) and now makes an excellent range of nut milks. They have recently started selling kombucha too, so definitely a brand to look out for.

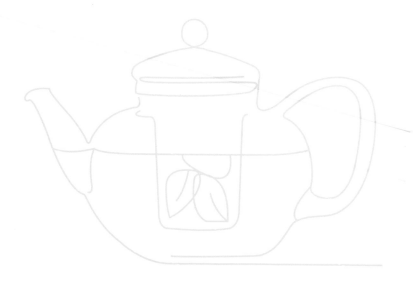

# WHAT TO DRINK INSTEAD OF RED WINE

One of the hardest things to nail if you're avoiding alcohol for any length of time is what to drink with food with which you'd normally drink a red – typically food from wine-producing countries such as France, Italy and Spain. You could, of course, experiment with de-alcoholized wine, but if you enjoy red wine, that's unlikely to satisfy you.

Soft drinks such as cranberry and other berry fruits are too sweet for a spag bol, lasagne or even pizza. They lack the acidity to stand up to a tomato-based sauce and the tannin to deal with rare meat (so they're no good with the Sunday roast, either).

## Red grape juice with balsamic vinegar

Cheap grape juice tends to be sweet, but a good organic grape juice like Biona could do the trick, particularly if you add a dash of balsamic vinegar (about 1 teaspoon for a small 125ml/4½fl oz glass works for me). The best option I've found with Italian food.

## Pomegranate juice

Again, avoid cheaper versions, or blend with beetroot juice (see page 150) to achieve a more wine-like flavour. It makes the beetroot juice – a bit of a Marmite drink – more palatable too. Good with Middle Eastern dishes – the sort you'd scatter with pomegranate seeds anyway.

## Elderberry juice

With more bitterness than most garden berries, it's the closest to a full-bodied red but can still feel a bit thick and syrupy. Dilute with a little still water.

## Sour cherry juice

Common in German and Eastern European shops, but also available in some health food shops and online, this has a touch of tartness that will stand in for pinot noir.

## Alcohol-free beer

Not exactly a substitute for wine, but it's worth learning to love the taste of alcohol-free beers if you don't already. A 0% porter is good with roast beef or a steak and mushroom pie, or try an IPA or pale-ale-style beer with pork.

# WHAT TO DRINK INSTEAD OF WHITE WINE

It's obviously easier to find a substitute for white wine than red. Just think of the flavours in white wine – citrus such as lemon and grapefruit, orchard fruits like apples and pears, and summer fruits such as peaches, nectarines and melons. The challenge again is to find drinks that aren't too sweet, particularly if you're eating seafood. It's the crisp dry whites, such as Chablis or Albariño, that are hardest to replicate.

### Chilled sparkling water
Might sound dull but with ice and a slice (of lemon) it's perfect with raw shellfish.

### Homemade lemonade
Not too sweet - the **Bergamot Lemonade** on page 44 would be perfect. Lime-based drinks such as the **Kaffir Lime Mojito** (see page 67) or an agua fresca (a fruity one rather than the floral one on page 170) are great with Mexican food.

### Elderflower cordial
A good alternative to Sauvignon Blanc.

### White grape juice with a splash of verjus
Just as with the red grape juice, you need a corrective dash of vinegar or, better still, verjus.

### Kombucha
Probably the drink I turn to most often with food when I'm not drinking, preferably plain rather than fruit-flavoured.

### Alcohol-free white "wines"
They don't really do it for me, but they're better than reds. See the list on page 183.

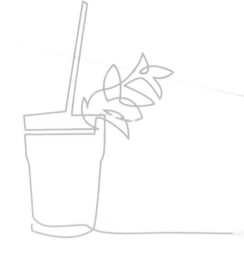

# WHAT TO DRINK...

### ...FOR A CELEBRATION

Bubbles are synonymous with celebrations, but what do you do if you're not drinking Champagne? To be honest, alcohol-free sparkling wine still has a way to go, especially if you don't have a terribly sweet tooth. The best option, I think, is to turn your bottle of alcohol-free fizz into a bellini with a dash of homemade (or good shop-bought) fruit cordial. Or there's always elderflower bubbly which looks suitably celebratory if you serve it in a Champagne glass. If the occasion is a romantic one, you might want to serve a **Passionate Lady** (see page 63). I also love the **Strawberry "Pimm's"** (see page 80).

### ...AS AN APERITIF

One of the trickiest times of day to handle is that after-work moment when you'd normally reach for a glass of wine. You feel you deserve a drink – and you do – but it doesn't have to be an alcoholic one. Nor should it be particularly complicated, but it should look – and taste – like a proper drink. If you're a gin and tonic fan, I suggest the **NG&T** (see page 91), the **T&T** (see page 176) or a **Double Lime and Soda** (see page 70). And if you like bitter Italian-style aperitivos, try a Crodino, Monte Rosso or the new Aecorn range (see page 184).

### ...FOR BREAKFAST OR BRUNCH

The great thing about alcohol-free drinks is that they're a guilt-free way to kick off the day – even as early as breakfast time. Smoothies or shakes like the **Strawberry Sunrise** (see page 154) and **Frozen Raspberry, Coconut and Chia Shake** (see page 140) will get you off to a healthy start or, to pull out the stops for a brunch, show off with a **Breakfast Martini** (see page 54) or a **Classic Virgin Mary** (or any of the "Marys", see pages 84–89).

## ...ON A SUMMER'S DAY

Undoubtedly the easiest time of year to get into the AF habit – it could almost make you give up booze for good. So many of the recipes are perfect for summer. Here are some of my favourites:

Gooseberry and Elderflower Cordial (see page 36)
Frosé (see page 106)
Fresh Strawberry and Watermelon Margarita (see page 58)
Kaffir Lime Mojito (see page 67)
Croquet (see page 83)
Bergamot Lemonade (see page 44)
Lemonade and Ginger Beer Shandy (see page 70)
Citron Pressé (see page 160)
Long Island Iced Tea (see page 71)
Piña Colada (see page 74)
Mai Tai (see page 78)
White Sangria (see page 105)
Lavender Milk (see page 138)
Iced Coffee Shake (see page 136)

## ...ON AN AUTUMN EVENING

As the nights draw in you may need a little bit more comfort drinking. It's also a good opportunity to make the best of the harvest. Try the Blackberry and Cinnamon Shrub (see page 48) or the beautiful pink-gold Quince, Honey and Lemon Cordial (see page 34). And two great drinks for Halloween and Thanksgiving: Mulled "Cider" with Roasted Apples (see page 102) and Spiced Pumpkin Latte (see page 131).

## ...ON A WINTER'S NIGHT

There's nothing like wrapping up on the sofa with a good book and a hot toddy, but give it a twist with turmeric to make an on-trend Golden Turmeric Tea (see page 171). More indulgently, you could make yourself a mug of Red Wine Hot Chocolate (see page 100), or a sophisticated Chocolate Espresso Martini (see page 92) for an after-dinner treat.

## ...AT CHRISTMAS

What would Christmas be without mulled wine? You'll be pleased to know its non-alcoholic equivalent (see page 99) is equally delicious. Or rustle up a festive red cocktail from an easy-to-make fresh Christmas Cranberry Cordial (see page 32).

# BEST BETS AT THE PUB

Pubs are not the worst places to find an alcohol-free drink, but the choices can be limited and the boozy atmosphere intimidating. But things are rapidly improving. I had a delicious blood orange and turmeric drink in a can (from Nix & Kix) in a far from fashionable pub in London the other day. And the gin boom has meant that most pubs have a good range of tonics and a proper amount of ice (remember those G & T's when they grudgingly dropped one cube into the glass?). The alcohol-free beer boom has also meant there should be something for non-drinkers and drivers, especially in country pubs, even if it's only a big name lager like Heineken. And more and more local breweries are brewing their own.

Here's how to mingle in with the crowd...

### Tonic with ice and lemon
Passes for a G & T. In smart pubs you may even get a choice of tonic. Or even a slice of lime or pink grapefruit.

### Ginger beer shandy
Ginger beer and lemonade. Make sure they understand it's ginger beer, not beer. Or ginger beer on its own at a pinch.

### Alcohol-free beer
All the big brands like Heineken, Beck's and Erdinger do AF lagers these days. I personally prefer Peroni if it's on offer – and you'll find Brewdog's Nanny State in Brewdog bars.

### Alcohol-free cider
Ideally made by a mainstream cider-maker like Sheppy's, rather than a fruit cider which tend to be more tailored to soft drink lovers than cider fans.

### Virgin Mary
Depends on the pub, but most should be able to rustle up a tomato juice and keep a bottle of Lea & Perrins handy.

### Lime and soda
Could easily be mistaken for a mojito, especially if you can persuade them to stick a sprig of mint in it.

# BEST BETS IN A RESTAURANT OR BAR

It may surprise you but you're more likely to find a good alcohol-free option in a swanky restaurant or bar – though you won't pay a lot less than you would if you were drinking. Many stock Seedlip (see page 184) or other alcohol-free spirits. "Mocktails" have also come a long way from the sickly concoctions (and silly names) that used to be standard fare. They're refreshing and sophisticated – I'll often order one in preference to a boozy cocktail even on a day when I'm drinking. And there's an increasing number of "dry" bars dedicated to alcohol-free drinks (see pages 202–203).

Many fine dining restaurants now offer alcohol-free pairings for their tasting menus, Noma in Copenhagen, Clove Club and Hakkasan in London and Eleven Madison Park in New York being four. Again, it's not a question of settling for second best – the drinks are often developed in the kitchen alongside and involve similarly foraged ingredients to the food. You definitely don't miss out.

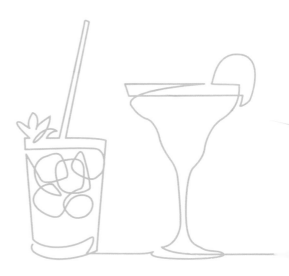

# WHAT TO DRINK WITH...
*Food pairing for non-alcoholic drinks*

One of the downsides of not drinking is that wine is such a natural accompaniment to food. Think of the Italian, French and Spanish dishes that you love and chances are you would normally have a glass of wine with them. This is not so much of a problem if you're just taking a day or so off the booze – you can happily eat something like a salad or a stir fry, with which you probably wouldn't drink anyway – but as a long term or even permanent situation it's more of a challenge.

Still, it's not as if there's any lack of alternatives, as I hope I've already demonstrated. It just needs a bit more flexibility in your thinking. And an understanding of some basic principles:

• It's more useful to think of the way a dish is cooked than the basic ingredient. So in the case of chicken, for example, think about whether it's roast chicken, a chicken salad or a Thai green curry.

• Is it a light dish – fresh, raw, crunchy, say – or a more intensely flavoured one like a Sunday roast or a barbecue?

• Are there sides or other dishes on the table to take account of whose flavour may dominate the plate? Sweet potatoes, for instance, will up the general sweetness of a meal.

The difference between wine and soft drinks in particular is that the latter tend to be sweeter, lighter (because of the lack of alcohol) and (with the exception of lemon drinks and vinegar-based drinks like shrubs) lacking in acidity. You miss out on tannin – the element of wine that goes so well with red meat – too. But if you're used to drinking beer or cider with your meal, you're in luck. There are many good alcohol-free alternatives.

If you're still struggling, the key is to think of the flavours that work with a dish, then reach for a drink that includes them. So, eating duck? Duck goes with cherries, so a cherry-flavoured drink (like the **Wild Cherry and Star Anise Cordial** on page 31) will be great with it.

Follow these guidelines for the main food groups, and see overleaf for the most popular cuisines.

## Beef and lamb

Check out the list of red wine alternatives on page 190 and the **Beetroot and Pomegranate "Pinot"** on page 150. Tomato juice (and Virgin Marys) pair well with rare roast beef and a steak tartare, especially the **Rosbif** on page 89. Coffee and Coca-Cola work well with burgers, as I'm sure you know.

## Pork and Chicken

White meats like these are often partnered with fruits like apples and apricots, so juices made with those fruits tend to work too, as do alcohol-free ciders. With fried chicken, try a root beer.

## Seafood

Perhaps unsurprisingly, water is really good with all kinds of seafood, especially raw or simply prepared shellfish. Personally I like sparkling water with a little ice or lemon, but it's up to you. With dishes with a touch of spice, make it coconut water or water kefir. With smoked fish try a **Kvass** (see page 120–121) or an alcohol-free lager. And look at the list of white wine substitutes too (see page 191).

## Salads and Veggies (especially greens)

Salads go well with vegetable juices such as beet and carrot juice. Also, if there's a fruity element in them, like a scattering of pomegranate seeds, pair with a complementary fruit juice like pomegranate juice.

## Cheese

Apple or pear juice are good all-rounders with a cheeseboard, but there are individual cheese matches which work particularly well: Try elderflower cordial (or the **Gooseberry and Elderflower Cordial** on page 36) with goat's cheese. Green tea, especially matcha is spot on too. Quince-flavoured cordials are perfect with sheep cheeses like Manchego (think membrillo), and blackberry or elderberry juice with a blue. And if you've a taste for those stinky cheeses and can handle strong flavours, try Pu'erh tea.

## Desserts

Again it's often a matter of thinking what flavours would complement a dish. Almonds and raspberries are great together, so why not serve a raspberry flavoured drink with an almond tart. Or a **Lychee Martini** (see page 56) with a pavlova. With desserts you can get away with chilled shots of fruit cordials without much, if any, dilution. Coffee is great with chocolate, as you know, but also with caramel and nut flavoured desserts like sticky toffee pudding. Bring the after-dinner coffee forward.

# WHAT TO DRINK WITH...

*Matching drinks to different cuisines*

The hardest types of food to match, as I've already suggested, are ones where wine is the traditional partner to a meal, especially French and Italian. The easiest are from countries where wine is not a traditional accompaniment to a meal: for example the Middle East, Mexico or Thailand. While we wait for the wine world to produce a de-alcoholized version that's as good as alcohol-free beer, here's what to drink with your favourite cuisine.

### Italian

Aperitifs such as Crodino are fine, but it's what to drink with a lasagne that's the problem. An AF amber ale is probably your best bet, or a glass of San Pellegrino with a dash of bitters.

### French

The French at least are big on cordials, though they tend to be a bit sweet. It may have to be a Perrier or a **Citron Pressé** (see page 160). Or an alcohol-free wine with a drop of vinegar or verjus to correct the sweetness.

### Indian

Mango juice or **Mango Lassi** (see page 142); **Banana, Coconut and Cardamom Lassi** (see page 141); **Chai Latte** (see page 128); AF lager.

### Mexican

**Hibiscus Agua Fresca** (see page 170); **Frozen Strawberry and Watermelon Margarita** (see page 58); **Tepache** (see page 122); **Michelada** (see page 106).

### Caribbean

**Speightstown Sour** (see page 75); **Switchel** (see page 45), **Piña Colada** (see page 74).

Chinese
Lychee Martini (see page 56); Oolong, Jasmine or sour plum tea; Bubble tea (see page 168); Ginger ale.

Japanese
Kombucha (see pages 116–117); green tea, especially with sushi. Matcha Latte (see page 132) goes well with desserts and cakes; Genmaicha tea.

Thai and Vietnamese
Ginger and Lemongrass Cordial (see page 186); Kaffir Lime Mojito (see page 67). Off-dry de-alcoholized wines like Torres Natureo muscat would work with Thai.

Middle-eastern/Turkish/Lebanese
Pomegranate juice; Apple and Saffron Sharbat (see page 159); other sharbats and shrubs; Rhubarb Cordial (see page 39).

Moroccan
Fresh orange juice, straight or mixed with Water Kefir (see page 114); Quince, Honey and Lemon Cordial (see page 34); Moroccan mint tea (see page 167), especially with sweet pastries.

Greek
Bergamot Lemonade (see page 44) and other sharp lemony drinks.

German/Polish/Northern European
Wild Cherry and Star Anise Cordial (see page 31); Kvass (see pages 120–121); Kefir (see pages 112–115.)

Spanish
Alcohol-free beers; Sangria (see page 105).

There are plenty of other suggestions for food and drink pairing on my website, matchingfoodandwine.com.

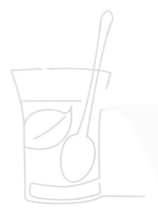

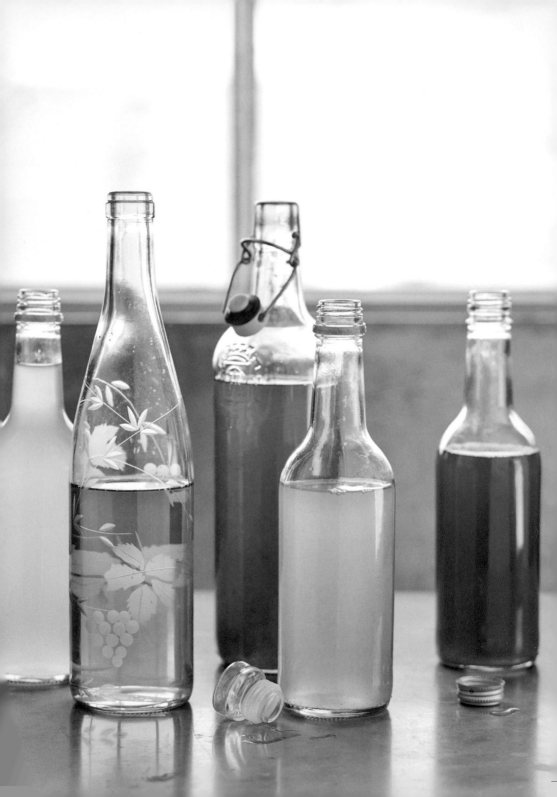

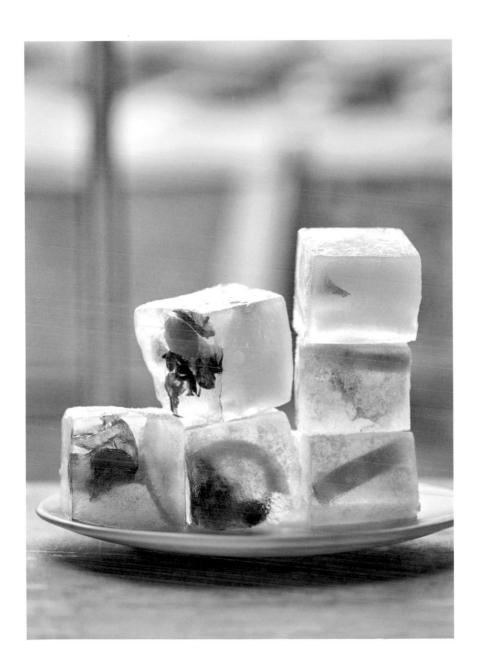

# Resources

The good news for wannabe non-drinkers is that there is not only an unprecedented number of alcohol-free drinks on the market but books, bars, websites, apps and social media support too. You absolutely don't have to be on your own on this journey

### Books
Some other books you may find useful that cover similar ground to this are *Dry* by Clare Liardet, *Redemption Bar* by Andrea Waters and Catherine Salway and *Seedlip: The Cocktail Book*, which also contain alcohol-free cocktail recipes.

*The 28 Day Alcohol-Free Challenge* by Andy Ramage and Ruari Fairbairns of One Year No Beer (see websites opposite) is a useful guide if you're embarking on Dry January or another alcohol-free month and, if you feel your drinking is verging on being a problem, read Catherine Gray's bestselling *The Unexpected Joy of being Sober*.

If you're serious about fermenting, you should buy Sandor Katz's definitive work *The Art of Fermentation* and/or *The Noma Guide to Fermentation*.

### Apps
As you'd expect you can easily track what you're drinking these days. Drinkaware tells you how many units and calories you're consuming and sets goals for drink-free days. I'm Done Drinking also calculates how much money you're saving.

### Instagram
Many of the authors, bars, brands and online communities I've mentioned also have Instagram accounts that are worth

following including Catherine Gray (@unexpectedjoyof), @joinclubsoda and @seedlip_ben (the founder of @seedlipdrinks). You might also want to follow @soberistas @sobergirlsociety, and @sobersommelier for day to day inspiration.

## Websites

There are a number of sites dedicated to selling alcohol-free drinks including the excellent drydrinker.com, which stocks bottles from all over the world, and zeroholic.co.uk.

There are also a number of websites that lend support to the newly sober including Club Soda (joinclubsoda. co.uk) which, runs regular mindful drinking festivals, the Australian website hellosundaymorning.org and oneyearnobeer.com, a subscription service which offers support and coaching when you take one of their challenges.

## Bars

A number of "sober bars" have sprung up devoted to alcohol-free drinks, among them Redemption Bar in London, which has branches in Notting Hill, Shoreditch and Covent Garden, The Brink in Liverpool and Café Sobar in Nottingham. The Virgin Mary, an alcohol-free pub, recently opened in Dublin. In the US there's Getaway in Brooklyn, Vena's Fizz House in Portland, Maine and The Other Side in Crystal Lake, Illinois.

There are also some fine dining restaurants that offer alcohol-free pairings (see page 195).

# Index

# Acknowledgements

Huge thanks to Joanna Copestick, my publisher at Kyle Books, for allowing me to write what I always hoped would prove a useful and timely book, and for providing me with such a fabulous team to achieve it: my long-suffering and lovely editor Tara O'Sullivan, copy editor Jo Richardson, designer Rachel Cross, and fabulous photographer Nassima Rothacker who, together with food stylist Becks Wilkinson and prop stylist Cynthia Blackett, is responsible for the stunning pictures in this book. And grateful thanks to my agent, Sarah Williams of Sophie Hicks, for dotting the i's and crossing the t's.

I owe a great debt to my neighbour Caroline Gilmartin of Every Good Thing for her expert advice and handholding on making kombucha and kefir, and fellow writer Kate Hawkings, co-owner of Bellita in Bristol, for an inspiring introduction to shrubs. And many thanks to the friends and neighbours who offloaded spare produce from their gardens and allotments to aid my multiple experiments.

I hope you all enjoy the results.